MOTORSPORT
Fitness
Manual

**To my parents for their interminable
support**
RSJ

**To the memory of Paul Hart, an incredible
man whose coaching philosophy inspired
many aspects of this book**
AB

First published in 2008

A catalogue record for this book is available from the British Library

ISBN 978 1 84425 543 6

Library of Congress control no. 2008926367

Published by Haynes Publishing,
Sparkford, Yeovil, Somerset BA22 7JJ, UK
Tel: 01963 442030 Fax: 01963 440001
Int. tel: +44 1963 442030 Int. fax: +44 1963 440001
E-mail: sales@haynes.co.uk
Website: www.haynes.co.uk

Haynes North America Inc.,
861 Lawrence Drive, Newbury Park, California 91320, USA

Page layout by James Robertson
Printed and bound in Britain by J. H. Haynes & Co. Ltd, Sparkford

Warning: Sports and emergency medicine is rapidly changing, with new
ideas and research conducted nearly every day. The author and publishers of
this work believe the content to be accurate and generally in accord with the
standards acceptable at the time of publication. However, neither the author,
the editors, Haynes Publishing nor any other party involved in the production,
distribution or sale of this work give any specific warranty as to its content,
and will have no liability for adverse results, inappropriate or excessive
use of the exercises and advice described or their level of effectiveness in
individual cases. All readers are advised to consult their fitness experts and/
or doctors prior to undertaking the exercises described as it is not intended
or recommended that this book be used as a substitute for medical or
professional advice.

MOTORSPORT
Fitness
Manual

Improve your performance with physical and mental training

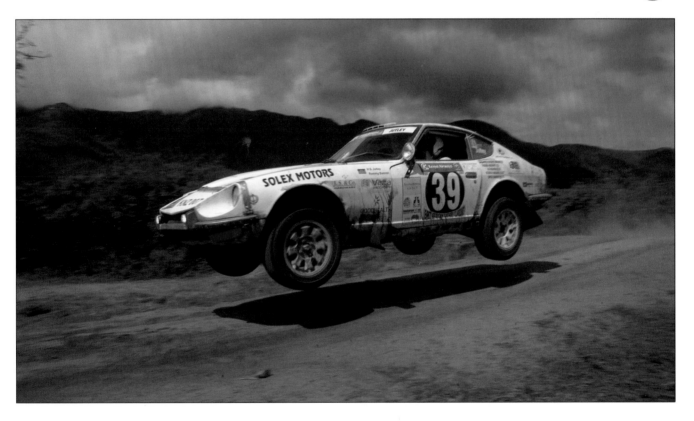

Dr R. S. Jutley BMedSci (Hon), MB, ChB, DM, FRCSGlas (C-Th)
Andy Blow BSc (Hon)

Forewords by Professor Sid Watkins MD, FRCS and Bernie Shrosbree
Contributions by Barbara Cox (Nutrichef), Chris Blythin, Mike Garth,
Dr Jonathan Whelan

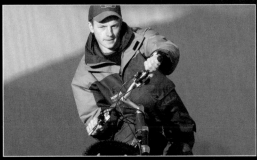
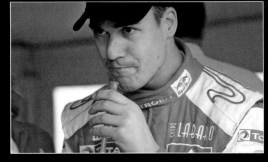
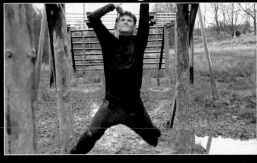
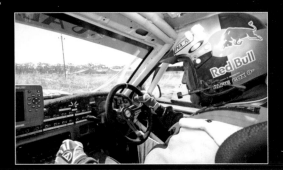

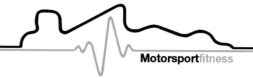

Foreword

by Professor Sid Watkins, OBE, MD, DSc, FRCS

President of the FIA Institute of Motor Sport Safety, 8 Place de la Concorde, 75008 Paris, France.

Dr Jutley has updated his very useful book which contained a great deal of information and excellent advice. The book, though primarily written to improve motor sport performance, is pertinent to many sports and activities and, indeed, to ordinary daily living.

In the splendid section on weight loss I found myself rechecking my height and weight and reached again for my calculator to determine whether I was obese or morbidly obese. In fact, to my relief, my Body Mass Index (BMI) at 26 placed me merely into the overweight variety. Having calculated my Resting Metabolic Rate (RMR), my daily energy expenditure and the necessary reduction in calorific intake in the first edition to return to my svelte and youthful figure, I have to report I have failed!

In the section on 'The event' extremely valuable guidance is given on diet and hydration. The maintenance of a sufficient fluid intake during performance in racing conditions with a high Thermal Load is of vital importance and is properly stressed.

Finally the new edition contains an updated section on emergency care in motorsport and on rescue which should be mandatory knowledge for the man in the street let alone motor sport competitors. There is a constant need to improve standards.

I once again enjoyed reading Dr Jutley's updated book very much. I am sure this pleasure will be shared with all of its readers, who will, in addition, acquire the knowledge to improve their own fitness and performance in life regardless of their vocations or occupations.

November 2008
Sabael
New York

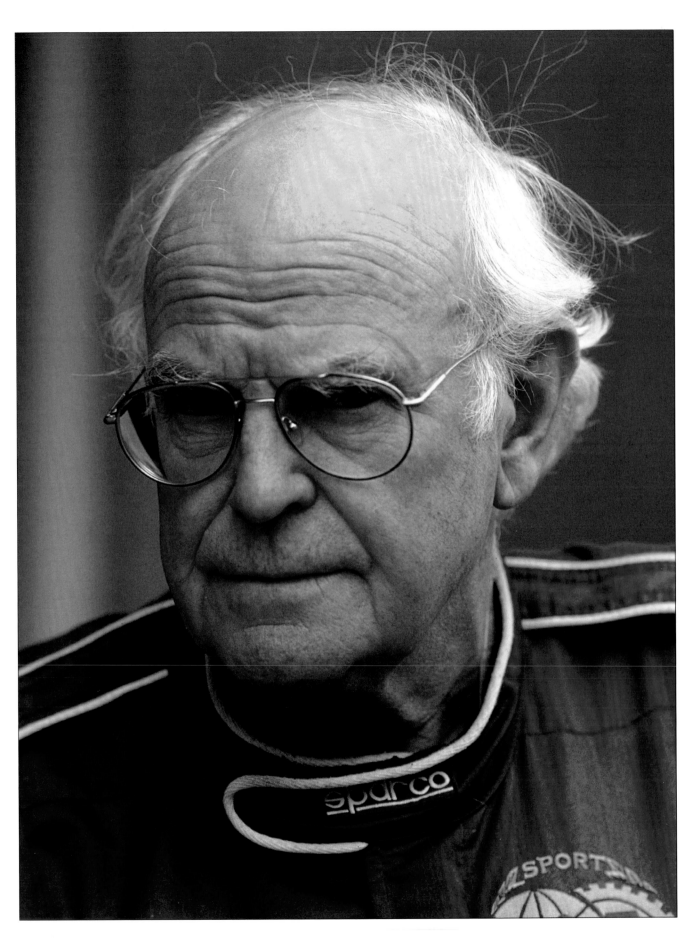

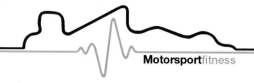

A few words by Bernie Shrosbree

I was delighted when Andy and Raj contacted me to contribute to the new *Motorsport Fitness Manual* after the substantial input I had into the previous book. Since my involvement with motor racing started in the early 1990s the focus on physical and mental preparation for drivers has increased massively, and this new edition certainly reflects the more modern and scientific approach now taken by professionals in this area.

I first met Andy as a graduate from the University of Bath and he worked under my guidance for several seasons in Formula 1 and World Rallying. In this elite environment his academic knowledge and practical experience as an athlete complemented my style of coaching and we became a strong team delivering top-level training and support services to a huge number of professional drivers. These days we still enjoy kayaking or biking together and chatting over our latest experiences and ideas about improving conditioning with innovative training. It is great to see some of this knowledge in print and available to competitors of all levels.

Dr Jutley's vast medical knowledge and enthusiasm for all things motorsport have impressed me since we first met many years ago. He has done a fantastic job in adding the results of new research to bring the book right up to date. By assembling a team of well-respected experts to add insight to each chapter there are now even more 'tricks of the trade' in here that will help any aspiring driver to reach a new level of fitness and preparation.

Finally, I would like to congratulate *you* on taking the first step towards improving your physical and mental condition for racing by picking up this excellent book. All it needs now is for you to have a read, then get up off the sofa and out training to put the theory into practice!

Bernie Shrosbree

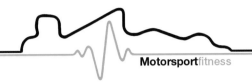
Acknowledgements

We are indebted to the many people who have helped us by providing their time, skills, and resources. This edition brings in many new contributors, and special thanks go to Chris Blythin, Philip Mosely, and Eliot Challifour for their ebullience; Barbara Cox of Nutrichef for her work on nutrition; Dr Jonathan Whelan for reviewing the chapter on emergencies, and Mike Garth for his work on Chapter 7.

We would also like to thank Dave Blow for his photography, Mike Gibbon and Anwar Sidi for new material, Nick Perry of Porsche Cars GB and Red Bull Photofiles for access to their media library, and R. K. Virdee and Louise Schrempft for their excellent illustrations.

Some contributors need no introduction: Mark Webber (Red Bull Formula 1), Dan Clarke (Champ Car World Series driver), Chris Pfeiffer (Streetbike Freestyle World Champion), Alan Kahn, and Bernie Shrosbree. We are particularly grateful to Professor Sid Watkins for once again providing his superb foreword and Lynne Sharpe for facilitating it.

My thanks also to the staff at Haynes Publishing, especially Mark Hughes for sharing our vision. We are also grateful to John Hardacre for his editing and Louise McIntyre and Flora Myer for managing the project. Finally, we would like to thank those who contributed towards the first edition whose material we have retained in the new book. Their names have been listed at the end of the book.

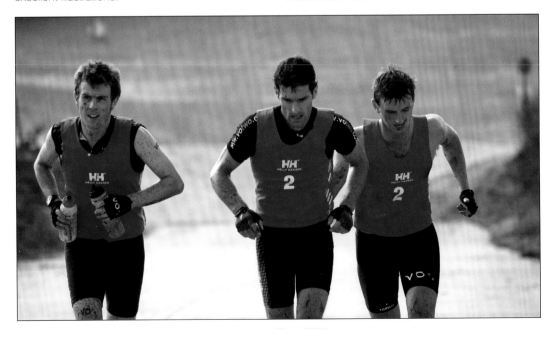

LEFT: Formula 1 driver Mark Webber is competing alongside the co-author Andy Blow and Eliot Challifour of votwo. *(Rob Howard of SleepMonsters.com)*

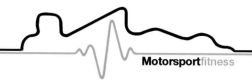
Introduction

Physical and mental fitness are now buzz words in just about every human pursuit, and it's no surprise, perhaps, that North America was quickest to spot the link between personal performance and fitness, not only in sport but also in everyday work. Indeed, it's not uncommon to find fully-fitted gyms and clinical psychologists readily available to staff in large US corporations – and, sure enough, productivity has increased.

It has long been realised, of course, that peak fitness is a prerequisite for a competitive edge in sport, but it could be argued that over the years most of those in motorsport have tended to ignore it. Even in Formula 1 racing, not so long ago, there were instances of drivers being exhausted and severely dehydrated, and quite often they would need help to simply get out of the car at the end of a race. Possibly the most memorable incident was Nelson Piquet collapsing on the podium at the Brazilian Grand Prix in 1982. In fact, that incident was probably what led FISA, motorsport's governing body at the time, to look seriously into driver performance and fitness. In motorsport, fitness is not just about driving faster, it's about driving more safely – about making fewer mistakes, which, at worst, could prove disastrous for the driver, other competitors and spectators.

Over recent years the fitness of their drivers has become increasingly important to the

RIGHT: Porsche strongly believes in driver fitness. Here, at a ten-day training camp in Fuerteventura, the works drivers are put through up to seven hours of intensive training a day supervised by Prof. Dr Frank Mayer. 'The combination of power training, various forms of endurance training, and team-building exercises has given my fitness level a noticeable boost', says Timo Bernhard from Germany, the reigning champion of the American Le Mans Series. *(ALMS)*

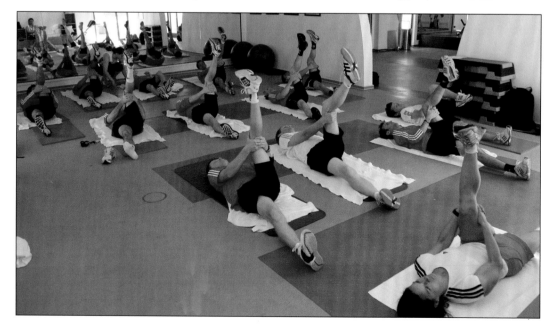

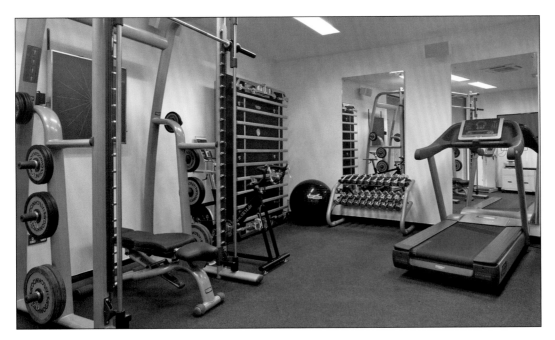

Formula 1 teams and top race/rally outfits, and they now routinely employ team doctors, physiotherapists, physiologists, psychologists, dieticians, and even ex-armed forces personnel to increase levels of mental and physical fitness. The Porsche Human Performance Centre at the Silverstone race circuit has facilities that would shame some of the best-equipped gyms. There's no doubt that the top drivers now have fitness levels comparable to top-class athletes. Sadly, though, the opposite is generally true for amateur competitors (hugely larger in number) who – like most of those living in developed countries – have a tendency to be overweight and in need of regular exercise. The race and rally cars available to them, on the other hand, are becoming more powerful and faster, and the competition tighter and fiercer. This combination is highly likely to lead to problems, and there are indeed problems.

Even amongst those competing in club and national motorsport events there are many instances of drivers being ill-prepared both physically and mentally. It's not unusual to see a driver make a fantastic start to an event only to fade as the day progresses, and the reason is usually that they are unaware of, or have been badly advised on, how to prepare for the event – for instance, about what particular components of fitness to concentrate on and how to develop the parts of your body most likely to be stressed during the event. This can lead to retirement from a race, or even crashing out – which is rather an expensive way of competing!

It is our own personal experience from competing at the topmost level, and our observations of the experiences of many other competitors that inspired us to write this book – the sequel to *Fit for Motorsport* published in 2003. We explain as clearly as possible the principles of training for fitness. Although the fitness industry remains one of the fastest expanding industries in the world there is a lot of confusion over terminology, training principles, and the basic concepts of fitness – and the innumerable websites set up by self-professed experts haven't helped. Many of their magic formulae for instant weight loss and miraculous fitness gains are based on poor scientific principles that can actually harm the body rather than achieve what they claim.

Motorsport Fitness Manual provides you with simple, established, and safe training principles. It is not a substitute for skill, so it is not designed to make you into a Lewis Hamilton, a Sebastian Loeb or a Mark Webber, but it will give you an insight into how they train and prepare for their races. Our aim is not to show you how to drive but how to maximise your driving by preparing yourself better both mentally and physically. Each chapter deals with a particular aspect of fitness and gives motorsport-specific advice on how to assess and develop it. There is also a chapter on emergencies, a subject which we consider an important part of any motorsport competitor's knowledge. Fortunately, emergencies are relatively uncommon, but when they do occur they can be very dramatic, and we provide an insight into what motorsport emergency procedures involve, so that if they do happen drivers are informed and cooperative with the rescue team.

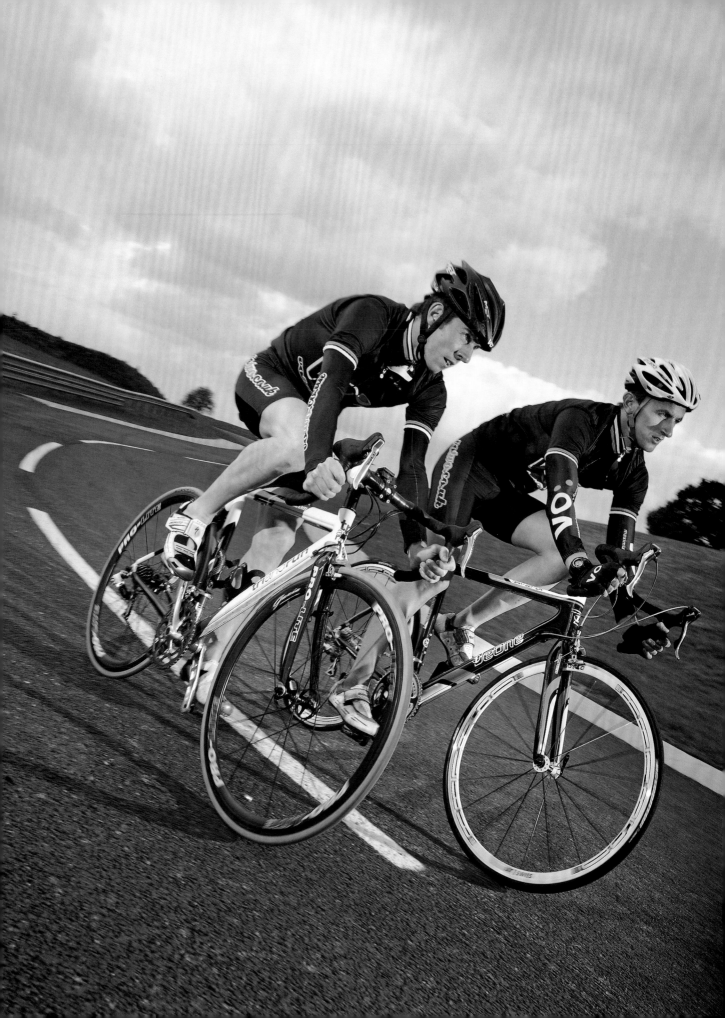

What is fitness?

We frequently use such expressions as fitness, shape, and conditioning when describing our physical and mental state, yet many would be hard put to define their exact meanings. Each relates to a perceived or measured state of body and mind and spans a wide range of ability, with top athletes (including top motorsport drivers) at the high end.

There are two important points to note about fitness. First, it can be measured. There are components to fitness (most easily remembered as the Ss of fitness – stamina, strength, suppleness, speed, skill, and spirit) and by periodic measuring of their levels we can see whether we are making any progress. Facilities, such as the Porsche Human Performance Centre based at the Silverstone race track in the UK, that specialise in the assessment and training of motorsport professionals, stand testament to just how seriously the industry is taking the subject of fitness and health these days. Second, fitness is highly sport-specific. For example, although Olympic weightlifters are extremely fit athletes, most would have difficulty running a marathon. The expected contribution of each component, and the training time dedicated to it, depends on the type of sport and the level of competition. There is, however, some degree of compensation between the components – an experienced squash player might use his or her *skill* to overcome younger opponents of greater *stamina*.

In 1998 I drove in my first Safari Rally, a round of the FIA World Rally Championship, and I felt that I was pretty fit, having climbed to the summit of a 20,000ft mountain in record time only months before. I paid little attention to preparing myself for this arduous race over three days, covering 2,500km in temperatures often around 30°C, and on the third stage, some 600km into the first day, I was time-barred for not finishing within the allocated period. The reason was simply that I was physically and mentally fatigued, and suffering from dehydration from my failure to plan my fluid and food intake. I learnt from these mistakes, and since then my participation in subsequent races, although as tough as ever, has been a thoroughly enjoyable experience. Dr R. S. Jutley

The components of fitness

■ **Stamina**. Arguably the most important component in any sport of significant duration is stamina, or endurance. In motorsport this component allows the competitor to perform prolonged sub-maximal activity without fatigue. Stamina should certainly never be ignored in any motorsport training programme. Also known as aerobic endurance, this component dictates for how long your body can undertake continuous physical work without tiring. Training for endurance is also very good for the human body from a general health perspective; having the potential to radically reduce the incidence of heart disease and other illnesses that have become major killers in the western world.

■ **Strength**. This component refers to the ability of the muscles to generate force against a resistance. Hence, strength training is often

OPPOSITE: Cycling is very often a favoured method of aerobic training for motor racers. Here co-author Andy Blow (left) is clocking up some miles on the Porsche Driving Experience tracks, Silverstone. *(Jonny Gawler)*

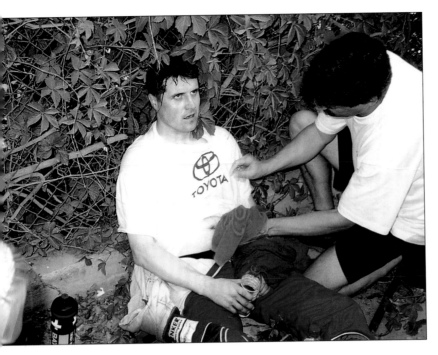

referred to as resistance training. Strength is critical in very specific areas for the motor racing driver, including the trunk and upper body. It is therefore of great importance that any strength-training programme seeks to highlight these body parts in order to improve performance, comfort, and safety when competing.

■ **Speed**. Speed refers to the rapidity of movement of the body, including reaction time and, to a certain extent, accuracy of motor control. Absolute speed is a priority for track athletes and in any sport where short and repeated sprints are necessary. In motorsport, however, it is quick responses, fast feet and rapid hands that count, rather than the ability to move the whole body swiftly.

■ **Suppleness**. Suppleness, or flexibility, refers to the range of motion that is available around joints of the body. In motorsport, suppleness is usually important to allow a driver to be comfortable and secure in the driving position they occupy, without having to constantly operate at or near the end of any joint ranges of motion. Occasionally, suppleness can be important if the worst should happen, as the 1990 Ladies World Rally Champion Louise Aitken-Walker found out. It was her flexibility that allowed her to extricate herself from the cockpit and roll cage to swim to safety when her car plummeted down a 150ft cliff during the Portugal WRC Rally and came to rest upside down and underwater in a 20ft deep river.

■ **Skill**. Skill and coordination are strongly linked and highly specific to the task. They refer to the smooth and accurate flow of movement as a task is undertaken, with top performers often credited with making a complex task appear effortless owing to the high degree of skill they possess.

■ **Spirit**. If the mind is ill-prepared, the body will perform poorly, and conversely a positive mental attitude can coax out the best possible performance on the day. This often underrated component of fitness refers to the valuable input of psychology in any sport. The well-worn saying, *'What the mind can conceive, the body can achieve'*, conveys this idea very well indeed.

Fitness in motorsport

The McLaren facility at Woking has a Human Performance Laboratory designed to improve and measure the fitness of their drivers. The VO_2max,

RIGHT: In any competition, the will to win or do one's best is by far and away the most important factor – motorsport is no exception to this rule. Hence 'Spirit' has the highest rating. 'Stamina' and 'Strength' are also massively important, and this is reflected by their equal proportions in the chart. 'Speed' and 'Suppleness' both play a part, and their contributions, whilst marginally less significant than some of the others, should never be overlooked. 'Skill' has been excluded on purpose as the book does not teach you techniques of driving.

Pie chart of fitness components

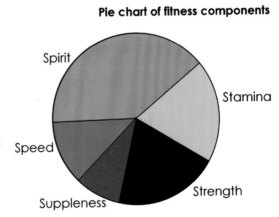

anaerobic threshold, and resting heart rates are all assessed at regular intervals during the year using state-of-the-art Technogym equipment. Similarly, at Renault F1's Human Performance Centre, drivers are assessed regularly throughout the year to ensure that high fitness standards are maintained. Tests include lactate threshold, VO_2max, motor reaction and fatigue reaction times, muscular endurance, and strength. Programmes are tailored to individual drivers to ensure they work on areas which need attention and not just what they enjoy doing. For instance, Fernando Alonso will favour different sessions from Nelson Piquet, but both have to work on areas identified in testing as needing improvement.

There is no doubt that most current top motorsport drivers are high-level athletes. Ask any trainer looking after the big-name competitors and they will tell you of the long months spent working on the various components of fitness. Bernie Shrosbree is well known amongst motorsport training circles. For many years employed by the Renault Formula 1 team as their Human Performance Manager, this former member of the Special Forces, and triathlete, is no stranger to physical and mental fitness. As a trainer of Jenson Button and Jarno Trulli, amongst other prominent personalities, such as the late 1995 FIA World Rally Champion Colin McRae, Bernie explains:

Although the various forms of motorsport require different specifics of fitness, for instance, strong neck and shoulders in F1 and strong lumbar region and forearms in rallying, there is a need for all drivers to have a base level of aerobic and strength conditioning on which to build these specific aspects.

Certain components of fitness are given more emphasis when it comes to motorsport-specific training. Apart from skill, which may be natural or developed, endurance, upper body and core strength are the most crucial components for motorsport competitors. Not only do drivers constantly battle with the steering wheel, often without the luxury of powered steering, they are also subjected to G-forces that place massive strains on their necks, trunks and upper bodies. In Formula 1 racing, G-forces as high as 4G have been reported during some of the corners at famous tracks. To subject untrained neck muscles to such forces could result in permanent damage. Impact G-forces during

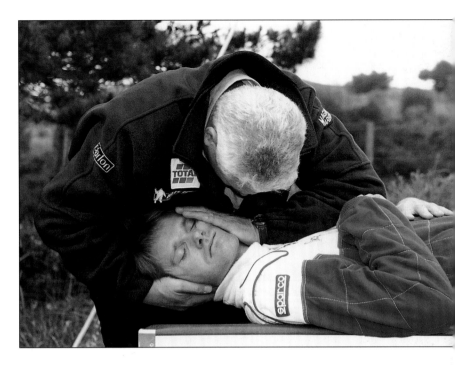

a racing accident can be astronomical, and a strong body is much more likely to withstand them than a weaker one. Also, should any injuries result from a crash, rehabilitation is always faster and more complete for those starting with a high level of strength and conditioning. The long duration of races, sometimes in hot and humid conditions means that anyone under-prepared, in terms of endurance, runs a constant risk of fatigue and exhaustion hampering their performance.

Dan Clarke (Champ Car World Series driver) explains...
People don't realise how hard it is on your body to drive a race car at 200mph. They also don't realise how fast your mind has to work to be constantly absorbing all the information of corners, other cars, and hazards that are approaching you at 200mph! Most people can probably handle this mental demand with practice. But if you're not race-fit and comfortable in the car running a two hour race, then you'll fatigue at some point, and then one of those hazards will most likely catch you out.

Andy Blow on the importance of overall fitness for driving...
As motorsport technology improves, cars are getting faster and the physical demands placed on the drivers are increasing accordingly. Being in peak physical condition for racing has never been more important, and in the future it's only going to get tougher!

ABOVE: Marcus Gronholm, the 2000 and 2002 World Rally Champion and Peugeot driver, receives on-the-spot attention from medical staff during a round. Rallying places massive stresses on the neck owing to G-forces encountered during acceleration and braking. *(Maurice Selden, Martin Holmes Rallying)*

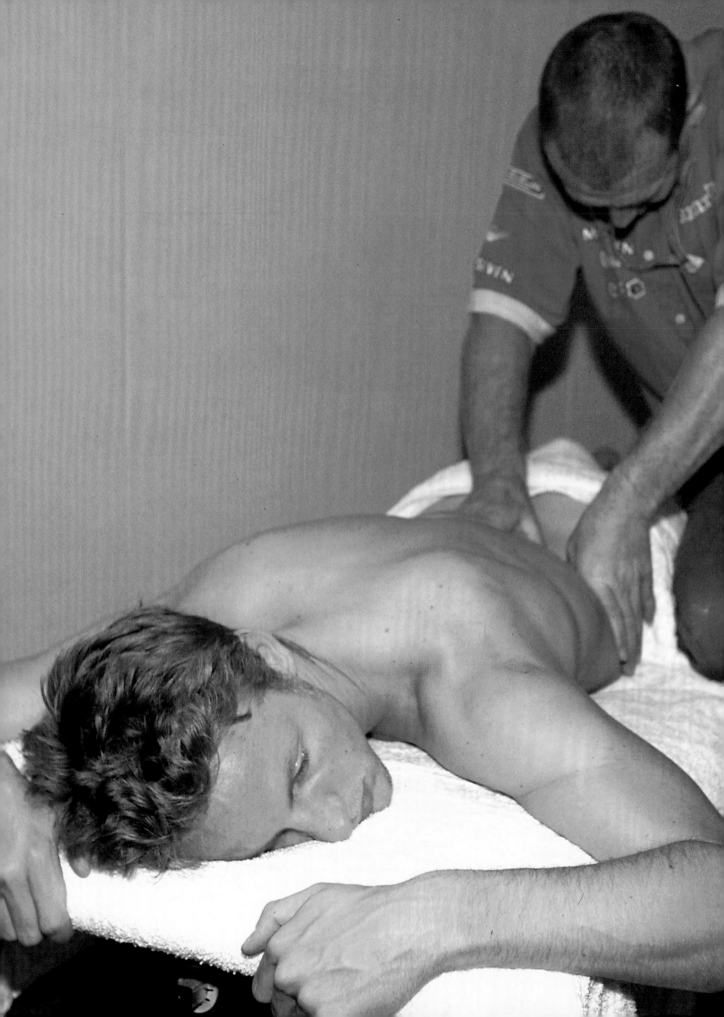

Before you start training

To maximise your performance and reduce the risk of damage to your body, it is essential that you incorporate two important routines into every training regime. These are *warming up* and *cooling down*. Ignore them at your peril!

Warming up

A warm-up means exactly what it says. It is a routine designed to elevate the temperature of your body to prepare it for what lies ahead. It increases the blood flow to your muscles and raises their working temperature. This makes the tissues, like your tendons (which join muscles to bone) and ligaments (which join bone to bone) more flexible, and guards them against strain and injury. Think of them as a piece of Blu-tack. If you stretch it when cold it will rip and tear, warm it up in your hands, however, and it will stretch many times over before breaking. An adequate warm-up also raises your breathing and heart rate and there is evidence that a warm-up prevents irregular heartbeats as the heart is stressed less suddenly. Finally, warming up allows time to prepare psychologically for the task ahead, be that through mental rehearsal, relaxation or increased alertness.

- Start gently and work your whole body so you feel warm. Suggested routines include brisk walking and/or light jogging, or any other whole-body activity, such as rowing. As a guide, if you work up a light sweat during the warm-up you are doing well. Avoid any explosive and sudden movements.
- Use warm-up techniques that are going to be replicated during your exercises. For example, do some flat terrain cycling for a mile or so if you are planning on a cycle ride. A brisk walk is a good start for running. In the gym, 5min to 15min on the rowing machine at low resistance is an excellent routine.
- DO NOT think that stretching is a replacement for warming up. It is now widely regarded that stretching is far more relevant as part of the cooling-down process and potentially even detrimental if used during warm-ups. Particularly tight muscles can be stretched after the main part of the warm-up if they need to be lengthened before training starts – a full stretching regime is not necessary, however.
- AVOID warming up more than 30 minutes before undertaking the training. A time lag of any longer will mean that your muscles will have cooled down considerably.

In cold conditions, wear adequate warm clothing to maintain muscle temperature when you have warmed up. The likelihood of pulling a muscle when running in shorts on a winter's morning is far higher than if you are wearing some running tights or jogging bottoms.

Cooling down

Just as important as easing into your exercise routine is easing out of it at the end. The benefits are several, yet a cool-down is largely ignored by many athletes, the preferred option being to head for the shower straight away. Remember that your body must adapt to its usual routine after the strenuous workout. It needs to re-synthesise and expel waste-products like lactic acid from

OPPOSITE: Just as important as warming up before training is cooling down afterwards, and here Jenson Button enjoys a massage to help in the cooling down process.

the muscles. It must prevent pooling of blood in places that no longer require high flow. Your heart must slowly regain its normal working rate.

A cool-down is done by gradually reducing the intensity of the exercise performed, or initiating a period of light activity, like walking or easy cycling. If on a bike ride, finish off by doing a few miles on the flat. On the gym machine, crank down the level of your training as you come to the end of your session. A whole body stretch is another excellent way of cooling down. There is some evidence that it prevents muscular soreness and stiffness. There is more detailed information on stretching in the chapter dedicated to flexibility. Other adjuncts to cooling down include the use of massage, warm baths, and jacuzzis. However, these come after the physical cool-down is finished and are not an alternative!

When warming up is not always the best strategy

There are times when warming up for training or competing is not such a good idea – specifically when you are operating in an extremely hot

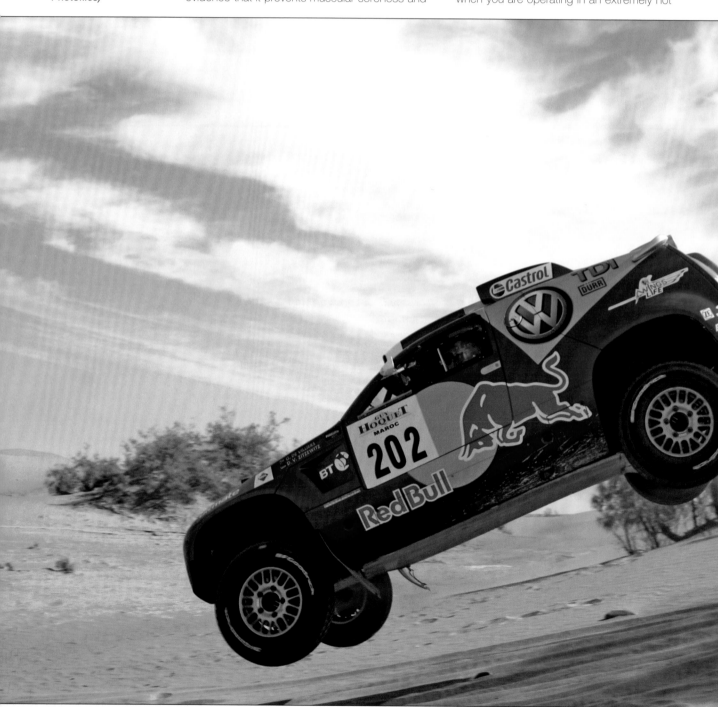

environment. On such occasions the muscles are often at or near their optimum working temperatures at rest, and one of the biggest challenges the body faces at such times is, in fact, keeping its core temperature down. In these circumstances 'warm-ups' should be kept very light with the aim of simply mobilising the joints that will be used in the exercise to follow. Preferably they should be performed in the shade and with adequate fluids and light, loose clothing to minimise any increase in core temperature. In recent years, research has been conducted into the effects of pre-cooling to lower core body temperature using special clothing or ice baths, a strategy which has been shown to be successful on some occasions. The specialist kit, which includes ice vests and cooling chambers, that has been trialled for pre-cooling is often very costly and out of reach for most amateur competitors. However, there are some basic strategies that anyone can employ prior to training or competing in the heat. These include:

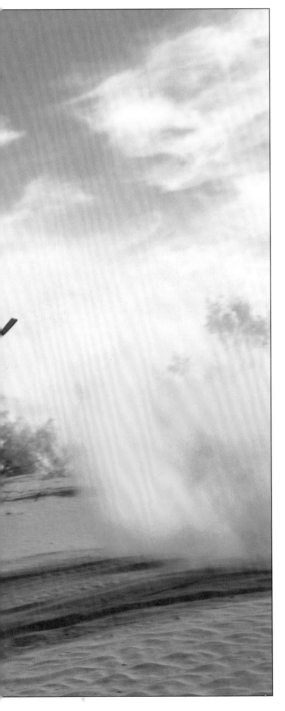

- Staying in cool or air-conditioned environments for as long as possible prior to starting
- Wearing loose, light-coloured clothing that covers most of the body (head especially) to reduce absorption of heat from direct sunlight
- Staying well-hydrated by consuming adequate quantities of cool fluids
- Keeping unnecessary physical exertion to a minimum.

Likewise, once racing is over in hot environments, the emphasis should be on reducing body temperature and rehydrating as soon as possible. Cool showers or baths and minimising exposure to the sun are sensible precautions, particularly if your schedule involves repeated stages or events in close succession, to avoid a gradual build-up in core body temperature over time.

Andy Blow on warming up before competition...

Motorsport competitors are always well aware of the need to warm up the engine, tyres, and brakes in order to optimise their performance in a race; no-one expects to come out of the garage at full revs and be straight on the pace. It's exactly the same for your body and mind, so practise different warm-up strategies for yourself to find out what works best as you prepare for training and competing.

References

Kay, D., Taaffe, D. R., Marino, F. E. 'Whole-body pre-cooling and heat storage during self-paced cycling performance in warm humid conditions', *Journal of Sports Sciences*, 1999; 17(8):937-944.

McMorris, T., Swain, J., Lauder, M., Smith, N., Kelly, J. 'Warm-up prior to undertaking a dynamic psychomotor task: does it aid performance?' *J. Sports Med. Phys. Fitness*, 2006;46(2):328-34.

Woods, K., Bishop, P., Jones, E. 'Warm-up and stretching in the prevention of muscular injury', *Sports Med.* 2007;37(12):1089-99.

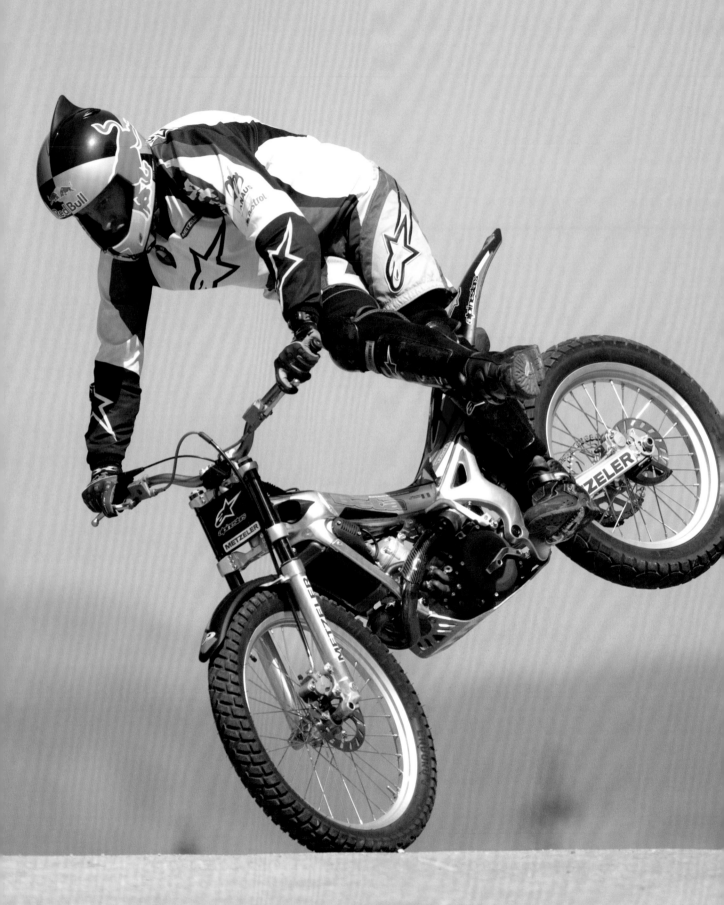

3

Stamina

To perform any exercise your muscles must be supplied with energy. This energy comes largely from the breakdown of fat and carbohydrate, a process which requires oxygen and is known as aerobic metabolism. Your capacity for continuing strenuous activity for any length of time, or your stamina, is therefore largely dependent upon how well your lungs and cardiovascular system work. As exercise intensifies, oxygen demand increases proportionally, and to meet that demand your lungs are called upon to breathe more heavily and your heart to pump

more rapidly to get the extra oxygen into the bloodstream and delivered as quickly as possible to the muscles you are using. How effectively this challenge is met is a measure of your fitness, but sooner or later there comes a time when the oxygen supply cannot keep up with the working demands of the muscles, and you become fatigued or exhausted.

As oxygen demand begins to outpace supply, your muscles will start to switch to anaerobic metabolism (burning fuel without oxygen). With anaerobic metabolism your muscles will operate

OPPOSITE: Chris Pfeiffer, Stuntriding Indoor World Champion, illustrates exceptional control on his bike. Chris works on his stamina by cycling regularly on his mountain bike or cycling machine. *(Predrag Vuckovic/Red Bull Photofiles)*

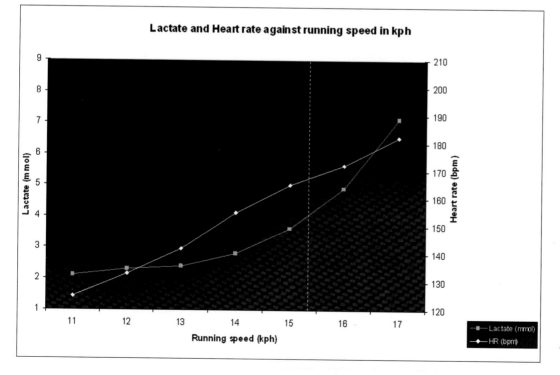

LEFT: The relationship between aerobic and anaerobic metabolism is demonstrated concisely by Dan Clarke, Champ Car World Series driver. The chart shows that as exercise intensity rises, and oxygen demand outstrips supply, he switches to anaerobic metabolism at the point shown by the dotted line. *(votwo with permission from Dan Clarke)*

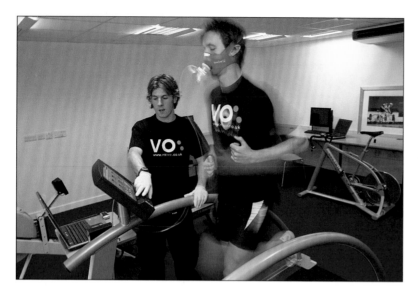

ABOVE: VO₂max testing involves analysing inspired and expired air to assess oxygen consumption as a measure of aerobic fitness.

Aerobic endurance is as important in motorsport as it is in any other sport. During competition, a driver's upper body muscles, especially, are constantly working to keep the car on the road. In endurance racing it may be several hours before a driver's muscles are allowed to rest, and during this time he or she will also be fighting the ongoing battle against dehydration in a high-temperature environment. If not conditioned beforehand, the working muscles will become prematurely fatigued by a rapid accumulation of lactic acid. Nearly all of the top racing teams now conduct regular physiological assessments of their drivers to keep track of their aerobic fitness levels. Whilst they utilise specialist sports science labs to do this, there are more accessible ways in which you can measure your own levels. The following section shows how to accomplish this.

about 19 times less efficiently than with aerobic metabolism and there will also be a more rapid build-up of lactic acid (lactate), which adversely affects muscle function and causes that unpleasant burning sensation. Training will bring about changes in your muscles at cellular level and can improve both your aerobic and anaerobic capacity.

The need for training to build up stamina is borne out by the results of research work conducted some years ago with Formula 1 and production car racing drivers. Jean-Louis Schlesser was found to have recorded a heart rate of up to 195 beats per minute in a

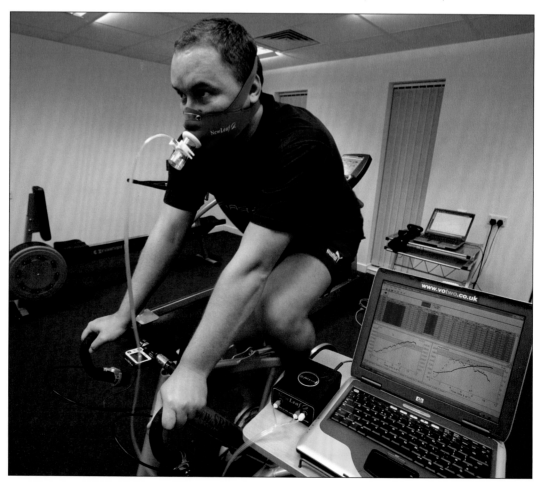

RIGHT: The most accurate method to assess VO₂max involves wearing a mask or mouthpiece to collect expired air whilst exercising at increasing intensity.

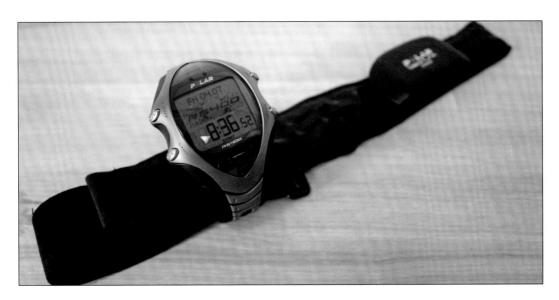

LEFT: Heart rate monitor.

production car race, and during a first session at Le Mans, Didier Pironi clearly showed a marked variation in heart rate between straights and corners. His heart rates were generally higher during cornering. More recently, Renault conducted their own research into this during Formula 1 testing at Valencia and Barcelona. I was involved in assessing some of the results of the study along with Bernie Shrosbree during his time at Renault F1. As with previous work, high heart rates were recorded – likely to be caused by a combination of the physical stress of driving, the heat stress in the car, and the adrenaline associated with high speeds and competitive scenarios. Generally, heart rates during motorsport can approach a driver's maximum rate, and this can only be sustained by those who are physically fit. It is possible that anyone in poor condition could suffer a heart attack if subjected to such high pulse rates. Dr R. S. Jutley

For racing drivers the other compelling reason to work on aerobic fitness is the effect that it has on heat acclimatisation. When you exercise for long periods, the body's core temperature naturally rises (as it does when subjected to a hot environment such as that inside a car). By performing regular long aerobic training sessions, even in relatively cool climates, you prepare the body to dissipate heat more efficiently and cope better in the heat. The fact that aerobic exercise tends to reduce body fat levels also helps this, as fat is an insulator preventing efficient heat loss from the body. In other words, fit, skinny people cope better in hot conditions than unfit, fat ones! Bear that in mind if your racing involves trips to exotic locations!

Measuring aerobic fitness –VO$_2$max and lactate threshold concepts

Peak aerobic fitness relates to the body's highest rate of oxygen consumption. It is referred to in sports fitness circles as the maximum oxygen uptake or VO$_2$max. To provide a more accurate measure, VO$_2$max is calculated as the amount of oxygen taken up per kilogram of body weight per minute (ml/kg/min). Effectively this gives you something of an aerobic 'power-to-weight ratio.' To a degree, the higher your VO$_2$max the fitter you are, although remember that values are determined by age, sex, height, and weight, as well as level of fitness.

The most accurate method to assess VO$_2$max involves wearing a mask or mouthpiece to collect expired air whilst exercising at increasing intensity. This method is, however, usually restricted to sports science laboratories, but the alternatives given on the following pages have been shown

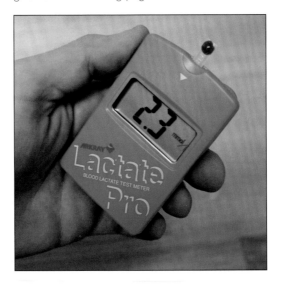

LEFT: Lactate monitor.

to correlate well with the more sophisticated tests. VO$_2$max testing may also be performed using treadmills and static bicycles, but these require special equipment usually found only in laboratories and some gyms.

The one-mile walking test – for complete beginners

Use this test if you have not been training. To calculate your VO$_2$max the figures you need are your weight in lbs, your age, the time you take to do the walk to the nearest 1/100th minute, and your heart rate at the end of it. The formula is:

$$VO_2max =$$
$$132.853 - (0.0769 \times \text{weight in lbs})$$
$$- (0.3877 \times \text{age in years})$$
$$+ (6.315 \times 1 \text{ for male}, 0 \text{ for female})$$
$$- (3.2649 \times \text{time})$$
$$- (0.1565 \times \text{heart rate at end of test})$$

Let's consider Jim, an amateur rally driver aged 35, weighing 85kg (187lb). He completes the course in 13 minutes 20 seconds (13.33min) and has a heart rate of 145 at the end. His VO$_2$max is then:

$$132.853 - (0.0769 \times 187)$$
$$- (0.3877 \times 35)$$
$$+ (6.315 \times 1)$$
$$- (3.2649 \times 13.33)$$
$$- (0.1565 \times 145)$$
$$= 45\text{ml/kg/min}$$

Remember to measure out an accurate mile and walk the course as fast as possible.

The 1.5 mile running test – for those with some recent training history

This is also known as the Balke test. Only attempt this test if you have been training beforehand and have a reasonable fitness level. Otherwise seek medical advice.

Measure out 1.5 miles and run the distance as quickly as possible. Then use the table to estimate your VO$_2$max.

Though VO$_2$max testing is an excellent

indicator of your general fitness level, in recent years the concept of 'Lactate Threshold Testing' has found favour with top athletes and coaches. This is due to the fact that once you have reached a reasonably high level of conditioning, VO$_2$max figures tend to stop improving, and any fluctuations measured do not necessarily relate directly to changes in performance. Lactate threshold (LT) refers to the point at which the body predominantly switches from aerobic exercise (with oxygen) to anaerobic work (without oxygen). LT is often referred to in terms of occurring at a percentage of VO$_2$max. As you get fitter, LT moves to a higher % of VO$_2$max, and therefore allows you to operate closer to your 'top end' for longer. The obvious advantage of this for drivers is that your 'comfort zone' for operating aerobically is increased, and therefore pushing harder for longer becomes possible.

Measuring your LT usually involves an incremental exercise test in a sports lab where heart rate and blood lactate levels are measured every 3-5 minutes. This test used to be very expensive and laborious but nowadays, with the advent of small and affordable lactate meters, many more gyms and sports coaches can offer the service. The Porsche Human Performance Centre based at Silverstone race circuit is one such place to offer this kind of assessment, with protocols specifically catering for racing drivers. In case you do not have access to such facilities, an alternative test is outlined below to allow you to estimate LT in relation to your heart rate. Bear in mind that this test should only be performed if you are very fit and confident of your ability to run at a consistently hard pace for 30min. You will also need a heart-rate monitor.

LT estimate test – only for the very fit

Warm up jogging for 10-15min. Then, on a level course, run for 30min at your very best even effort. A measured running track is the ideal place for this. Record your average heart rate for the final 20min of the run. If your monitor does not record average HR, make a mental note of it every minute or so during the final 20min to estimate the average. Record how far you ran.

Your average HR for the last 20min of the test is your estimated LT heart rate. You can use this figure to help determine your heart rate training zones, and also by repeating the test from time to time you can measure improvements in the total distance covered and see if your LT heart rate changes. As you get fitter you will find that you can run further and sustain a higher HR (and therefore higher % of VO$_2$max) for the 30min period.

RIGHT: VO$_2$max values in active people and elite athletes. The values generally peak in the third decade. With each decade the VO$_2$max declines by up to 10% depending upon the level of activity.

VO$_2$max values in ml/kg/min		
	Men	**Women**
Active	50-65	35-50
Elite athletes	65-90	55-70

Improving stamina – the training heart rate concept

It's clear that to improve your stamina you need to undertake exercise of a sufficiently high intensity, and that intensity is most easily measured by your heart rate.

Unless you have a heart problem, generally the lower your resting heart rate (pulse) the fitter you are. The method described is accurate when measuring progress in training and is used regularly by many athletes. Most individuals have a resting rate of between 60 and 90. With regular exercise your resting rate will drop as your heart becomes more efficient. Top marathon runners and some Formula 1 drivers have resting heart rates in the 30s and 40s!

To best take your resting rate, do it while lying still in bed having woken from a good night's sleep. This time is preferable as you are least likely to be subject to any influence from muscular activity or from the intake of stimulants such as caffeine in coffee or tea. The pulse at the wrist is ideal for measurement, or the carotid artery may also be used as described in detail in the emergency care chapter. Put your finger on your pulse and count the pulses over a minute. An easier way is to use a heart-rate monitor. These can be bought in most sports outlets.

Everyone wishing to train with a monitor should know their maximum heart rate. This number is important as it allows training intensity to be calculated. The most commonly used method for arriving at a rough estimate of your maximum heart rate is to subtract your age from 220. Jim, the amateur driver who is 35 years of age, should have a maximum heart rate of 220 – 35 = 185 beats per minute. Bear in mind that this is only an estimate, and whilst it fits with many people, for some it can be substantially different. To find your true maximum heart rate, having an incremental exercise test under the supervision of a qualified sports scientist or doctor is the best method.

Your training zone

Most experts recommend that to gain any benefit from exercise you should train within a particular training zone, usually between 50% to 85% of your maximum heart rate. This means that Jim would have a training zone minimum of 185 x 0.50 = 93 beats per minute, and a maximum of 185 x 0.85 = 157 beats per minute. Towards the higher end of your training zone your body tends to be close to its anaerobic threshold. Generally speaking, the fitter you are the more training you can do towards the upper end of your training zone without undue fatigue.

Time (min:sec)	Estimated VO$_2$max (ml/kg/min)	Fitness Level
Under 7:30	75	
7:31– 8:00	72	
8:01– 8:30	67	HIGH
8:31– 9:00	62	
9:01– 9:30	58	
9:31–10:00	55	GOOD
10:01–10:30	49	
10:31–11:00	46	AVERAGE
11:01–11:30	44	
11:31–12:00	41	
12:01–12:30	39	
12:31–13:00	37	FAIR
13:01–13:30	36	
13:31–14:00	33	
14:01–14:30	31	
14:31–15:00	30	LOW

The Karvonen formula

As mentioned previously, the '220 minus your age' method of establishing maximum heart rate is not particularly exact. A more accurate method is to use the Karvonen formula which takes into account your resting heart rate. It requires slightly more maths but is easy enough to work out. The steps are as follows:

1 Take away your age from 220.
2 Take away your resting heart rate from that value.
3 To work out the lower end of your training zone, multiply the result of Step 2 by 50% and add you resting pulse to it.
4 To work out the upper end of your training zone, multiply the result of Step 2 by 85% and add you resting pulse to it.

For example:
Jim has a resting heart rate of 80 beats per minute. According to the Karvonen formula his maximum heart rate should be 169, worked out as follows:

1 220 – 35 = 185
2 185 – 80 = 105
3 105 x 0.5 = 53; 53 + 80 = 133 (minimum training heart rate)
4 105 x 0.85 = 89; 89 + 80 = 169 (maximum training heart rate)

ABOVE: Estimation of VO$_2$max using the 1.5-mile running test. This is based on a population of males aged 20-29 years. By moving up one category, the values for females may be obtained. *(Used with permission from Fitness For Sport by Rex Hazeldine, Crowood Press.)*

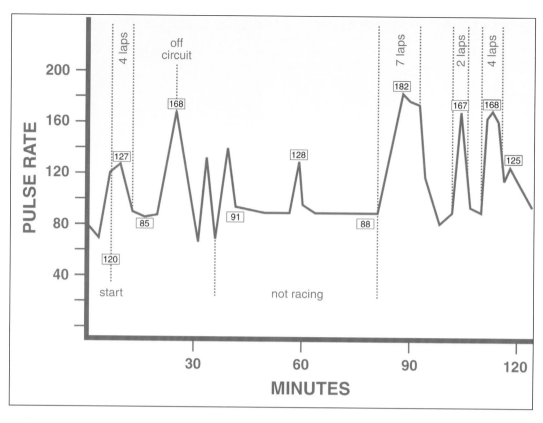

Why measure heart rates?

To some, measuring and calculating heart rates may sound tedious. However, it has been shown to be of great benefit when assessing progress during training. For example, you may find that Level 2 on the gym machine initially pushed your heart rate to 150. After a month the same level only raises it to 140. This shows a definite and measurable increase in stamina. Many elite athletes also use heart-rate monitoring to assess whether they have recovered from heavy workouts. If, first thing in the morning, their heart rate is higher than usual, it is likely that they have not recovered from their previous workout.

Another good indicator of improvement in fitness is the time it takes for your heart rate to recover to lower levels. Next time you are in the gym take your pulse rate as soon as you complete your training session, and take it again after a minute. Generally, the faster the drop the fitter you are.

Heart rate and perceived exertion – where training becomes an art and science

When training with heart rates it is important not to blindly follow the monitor, completely ignoring other signs of how hard you are working. Your RPE (rating of perceived exertion) is a way of assessing how hard you think you are pushing yourself. Many variations of this scale exist, with the Borg Scale (6-20 points) being the most prominent. The Borg scale, however, can be quite difficult to use, and specialist sports trainers use a simple six-point scale that is described below. Whether you are using a heart-rate monitor or not, it is worth asking yourself how hard you think you are working in relation to the scale, and then you can look at the benefits you should be getting from that session. As you become more practised with this over time you will get to 'know' your own body much better and optimise your training intensity to gain the desired effects. For instance, if you are very tired you may find that raising your heart rate up to the desired levels takes an unusual amount of effort. On those days it is best to throttle back and maybe even rest to aid recovery. If, on the other hand, you find that your heart rate zooms to high levels, with little sensation of effort and you are 'flying', you can limit how hard you are pushing to avoid overdoing it. Without doubt, the best method is to use a heart-rate monitor to guide your intensity and then fine tune your work rate by using the RPE scale. With sufficient practice you will become extremely proficient at doing this. After a long time many top athletes find that they are able to train almost exclusively on RPE, checking a heart-rate monitor just occasionally for reassurance that all is on track.

Modified Rating Of Perceived Exertion (votwo training zones)

VO$_2$MAX	All out exertion.	Not sustainable for any real length of time. Max duration 4 min.
Race Threshold (RT)	Race pace for short events up to 1 hour when well trained.	Mental and Physical battle to sustain pace. Max duration 1 hour for highly-trained athlete.
Lactate Threshold (LT)	Very hard, just under threshold sustainable to 2-4 hours max for well-trained athlete.	Athlete requires significant commitment and concentration to sustain intensity.
Tempo (T)	Strong aerobic training pace.	Athlete requires mental and physical focus to sustain intensity.
Base Endurance (BE)	Steady and controlled, minimal point to stimulate physiological adaptations to training.	The athlete perceives that work starts at this intensity.
Easy/Recovery (REC)	Very easy warm-up, cool-down or recovery.	Very gentle activity.

Descriptions of expected training effects in the six zones:

Recovery (Rec)	Work done in this zone aids the recovery process. It is done by training at a very easy pace, preferably on flat terrain. Benefits include increasing blood flow to the muscles to help remove muscle soreness, and reducing the free-radical build-up that causes muscle stress and damage. Active recovery at an appropriate pace leads to faster recovery than complete rest.
Base Endurance (BE)	Steady training at Base Endurance pace builds an aerobic energy system that will increase your endurance capabilities. Expected benefits include: increased size and strength in slow-twitch muscle fibres, increased stroke volume from your heart, greater economy and increased fat utilisation (especially during very long sessions). Base endurance pace generally feels comfortable, relaxed and can be sustained for long periods.
Tempo (T)	Tempo training is a more intensive workout than BE, but it still remains predominantly aerobic. It is ideally done in timed blocks, consistently paced and without interruptions. It offers similar benefits to training at BE, although as it is more demanding more recovery time is needed. Because of the increased intensity it is a very efficient way of training aerobically if time is limited. Other benefits of tempo training include better fuel utilisation during long races, increased capacity for more intense workouts, increased muscular endurance, increased muscle glycogen storage capacity, and improved aerobic efficiency. Tempo workouts require a high degree of concentration and commitment to complete properly.
Lactate Threshold (LT)	LT is most accurately determined in a sports lab. Training in sustained blocks around the intensity of your measured LT is a proven way to move this threshold to higher speeds. However, this type of training is demanding and needs to be balanced with plenty of recovery time to allow the benefits to show through. Usually one to three sessions per week focusing on this is enough. Spending progressively longer durations at intensity just below LT is an effective yet relatively safe way to achieve improvements in this area. After a phase of LT training, a reassessment in a lab to measure progression in this area will tell you how effective it has been.
Race Tempo (RT)	Race tempo refers to the intensity you can sustain for a race of approximately one hour in duration. As the RT zone spans a range of intensities, you may be able to sustain the higher ranges for shorter events and the lower ranges for longer events. Interval work at RT is a very powerful training tool if used with sufficient recovery to allow adaptation.
Maximum effort (Max)	Maximum effort refers to sustaining the highest intensity that you can for a given time period. Usually, this is only for a few seconds (to improve top speed and anaerobic capacity) and up to a few minutes (to improve lactic acid tolerance and increase VO$_2$max). Training at maximum capacity from time to time is required to push physiological and psychological limits to new levels.

Designing an aerobic exercise plan

Naturally, exercise plans are tailored to suit needs. These might be to burn fat, to lose weight, to gain weight, to build strength or to improve fitness and restore a feeling of well-being. Our aim here is to improve your fitness level, or in other words to improve your VO_2max and lactate threshold, and lower your resting heart rate. Bear in mind that having a very specific goal to train for is the best way to ensure the success of a training plan. Mark Webber organises a gruelling adventure race challenge around Tasmania every winter that has the dual aim of raising money for charity and focusing his training during an otherwise quiet time of the year. Consider choosing an event, race or other physical challenge to build up to alongside your regular racing and you will find much stronger motivation to get out and put in the hard work required to get really fit.

Training is all about getting the progression just right. Be sure to gradually build up the intensity and duration of your regime. It is important not to go at it too strongly and run the risk of injuring yourself early in the programme. A suggested routine is:

- Start off with three sessions a week with at least a full day's rest between sessions.
- Make each session variable in length and intensity. For example, go on for up to an hour at the lower end of your training zone. On other days, go for 40-minute sessions at up to 85% of your maximum heart rate.
- As your fitness improves, aim for five sessions a week.
- Increase the duration of the training by around 10% three weeks in a row, and then schedule in an easier week on the fourth for recovery.
- The intensity of your training will change automatically as you find it progressively easier to perform the same task.

To maintain and improve stamina, Jim Moodie (1999 TT standing start lap record holder) subjects himself to a fairly punishing routine in the gym, especially during winter months before the race season. Jim does not enjoy running, and maintains 80% of his maximum heart rate on the cross-trainer for up to 30 minutes before pushing himself to 100% for five minutes at the end of the routine. This should only be attempted by those who are exceptionally fit and capable of withstanding the stresses of the exercise.

A weight-loss programme generally requires longer workouts so the body burns fat preferentially. As a guide, 60min-plus workouts are needed at around 50-70% maximum heart rate (in the REC and BE zones) to make significant progress. If you can find activities that you enjoy doing for more than two hours, this is very beneficial as the body really starts to rely heavily on fat metabolism after this point. Try to work out regularly at this low intensity, but also intersperse the long sessions with some shorter ones at a higher intensity. This ensures that your top-end cardiovascular conditioning and LT development is not neglected. Remember that if weight loss is the main aim of your programme, then paying attention to good nutritional practices is essential. More details about this can be found in the nutrition chapter.

Modes of training

For the motorsport competitor, a good mixture of training modes is desirable for building aerobic fitness. This helps to keep the programme interesting and varied, reduce the chance of overuse injuries, and ensure good conditioning of all body parts. Start with activities that you are familiar with and enjoy, and then challenge yourself with a new sport from time to time. The classic exercises such as running, cycling, swimming, and using the CV machines in the gym can be complemented with rowing, kayaking, cross-country skiing, mountain-biking, climbing or whatever inspires you to get out training. Remember that training does not need to be a chore – it should actually be enjoyable most of the time, as Chris Pfeiffer (Indoor Streetbike Freestyle World Champion 2007 and Stunt Riding World Champion 2003) states:

Mainly I cycle regularly. At home I prefer my mountain bike, and whilst on the road I sit on the cycling machine in the hotels for half an hour per day. This is so important for several reasons: endurance is the basis for all my activity, it helps me to maintain concentration until the end of my ride and to recover faster. Also bicycling is very good for my stressed out knees. And, last but not least, I relax during my endurance training and feel really good and fresh afterwards. To achieve that, it's very important not to go too fast.

Maximising training

As your fitness improves, you can start to modify your training programme to include the following with a view to maximising the benefits.

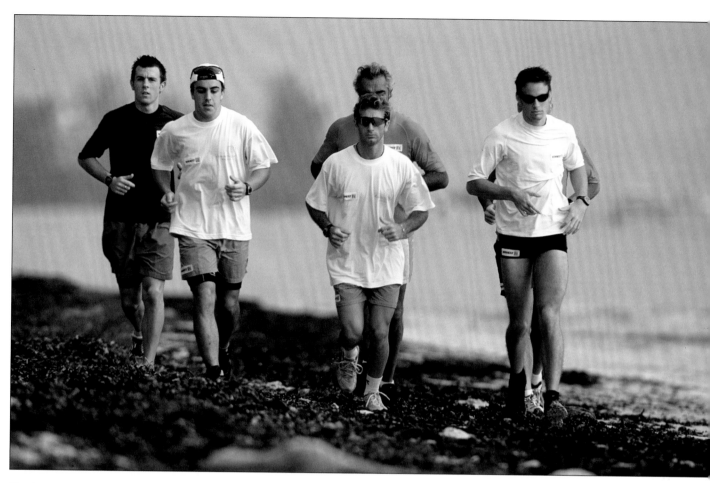

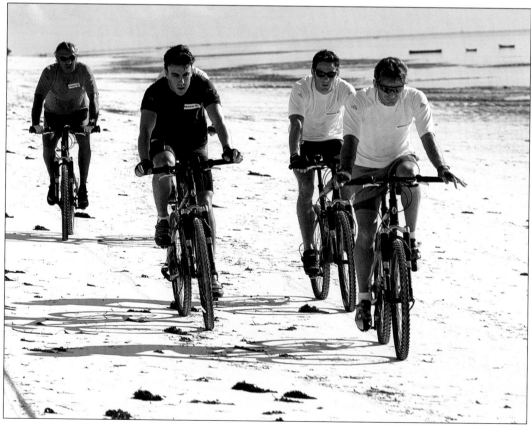

ABOVE AND LEFT:
Former Renault
F1 drivers, Jenson
Button, Jarno Trulli,
and Fernando Alonso,
during their driver-
training programme in
Kenya before the start
of the 2002 season.
The drivers are seen
combining cross-terrain
trekking and cycling
to maximise their
endurance. *(Renault F1)*

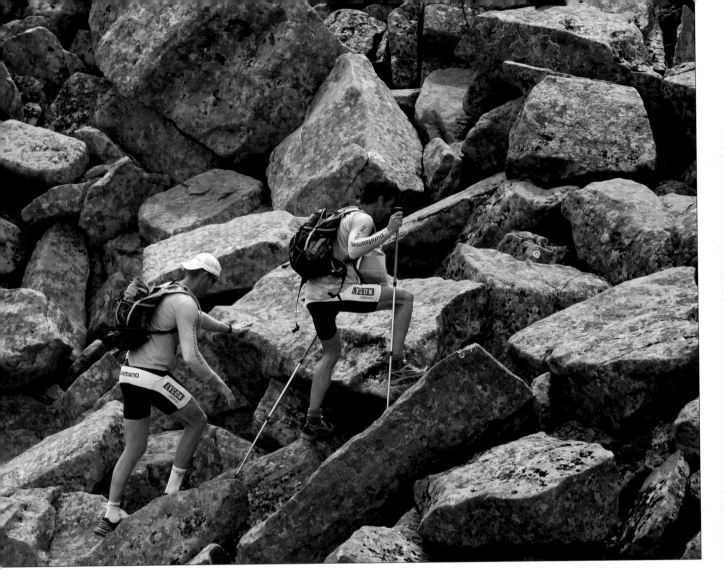

Fartlek

Swedish for 'speed play', this training method allows you to vary the pace and intensity of your programme at random and in a carefree manner. For example, when jogging decide to sprint for five seconds at every third telegraph pole and slow to a fast walk at every fifth for 100 yards. When starting out, try to push yourself into the LT zone on the RPE chart for short periods. As you get fitter, working into the RT and even VO$_2$max zones becomes possible.

Interval training

This is a very popular method of aerobic training where you combine short, intense spurts of exercise with short periods of recovery at lower intensity exercise. The spurts may last as little as 15 seconds or as much as 10 minutes. Many gym treadmills, cycle machines, rowing machines, and cross-trainers now offer interval training as a standard programme. The advantage of intervals is that it progressively builds up aerobic capacity in the muscles by taking them close to

their fatigue limit. It also breaks up long sessions into manageable chunks that relieve the potential boredom of training. Working in the LT zone at first, and later the RT and VO$_2$max zones, with active recovery periods between them is the aim.

Hills and off road training

Walking slowly up a steep hill requires as much energy as running on the flat. Walking on sand requires twice as much as doing the same on hard ground. Any mode of training done on rough or hilly terrain increases the energy output required, so adds significant value to the session. Ten miles of cycling on rough mountain tracks is very different from ten miles along a canal tow path, as you can probably imagine! Also, the psychological benefits of getting out of the gym and into the natural environment are very important and cannot be underestimated.

Circuit training

This is a widely used method to improve aerobic and muscular endurance as well as speed.

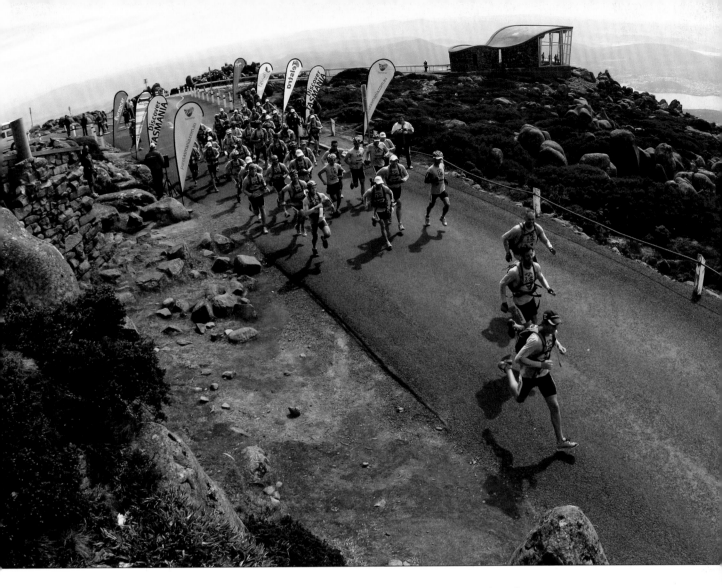

It involves setting up a circuit of aerobic and muscular exercises that may be specific to the sport. Details of motorsport-specific circuit training appear later in the book.

When to take a break

Just as important as training hard is knowing when to stop. Overtraining is a real problem for highly-motivated sports people, and occurs when you are not recovering sufficiently from the exertions of training and competition. If you experience the following signs then you have probably overdone it:

- You always feel tired and sore
- You are very prone to colds and minor infections
- Your sleep patterns are interrupted
- Your concentration span is short
- You are easily irritated
- Cuts and abrasions take abnormally long to heal
- Your appetite is poor
- You lose weight rapidly.

If you find yourself suffering symptoms such as those above, the first response is to take some time off from training. Ensure that you are eating well and staying hydrated. Usually 48 hours of recuperation is sufficient to recover from a mild dose of overtraining. If after that time you are still feeling below par then up to two weeks of time off can be required to fully recharge your batteries. Should a prolonged lay-off prove unsuccessful, then a visit to the doctor is the next step to rule out any illness or deficiency that may be causing you to underperform. Keeping a training diary, and ensuring that your training is gently progressive, including time set aside for rest and recovery, are two of the best ways to avoid overtraining from happening in the first place.

Andy Blow on training for aerobic fitness...

More than anything else, finding sports you love doing is crucial when designing your aerobic exercise plan. To get really fit, you'll need to spend many hours training, so you may as well enjoy it!

ABOVE: Each year, Formula 1 driver Mark Webber runs a gruelling adventure race in Tasmania which raises money for charity. It takes competitors through 350km of terrain with biking, trekking, and kayaking. *(www.gettyimages.com)*

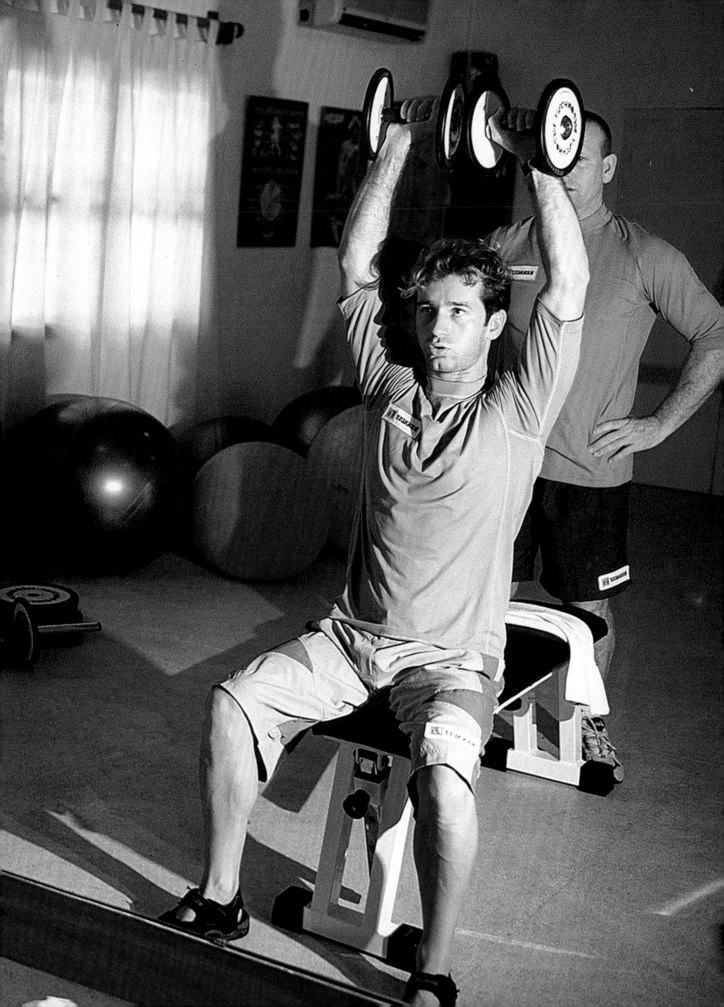

Strength

Strength is an extremely important component of fitness for the motorsport competitor, and this chapter gives specific advice on how to improve the aspects of strength that are critical for drivers.

Put simply, strength is a measure of the level of force that you can exert against a resistance. Hence, strength training is often referred to as resistance training.

In this chapter we are going to focus on two types of strength, isotonic and isometric. There are others, but these are the most relevant to driving. Isotonic (iso = equal and tonic = tone) strength is also known as dynamic strength and relates to the normal contraction of muscles as body parts are moved, for example, to lift a heavy weight off the ground. Isometric (iso = equal and metric = length) strength is sometimes referred to as static strength and relates to muscles exerting pressure without changing length. Here the muscle exerts a pushing force such as pressing straight-armed against a solid wall. Motorsport requires a combination of isotonic and isometric strength.

Forces of up to 4G or 5G are not uncommon during braking and cornering in motorsport during racing. Considering that the combined weight of an average head and helmet is around 4kg (about 9lb), this means the neck muscles must support up to 20kg (44lb) during such manoeuvres. A typical track event lasts over 50 laps, each with around 12 corners, in heat and humidity that drains away the energy of any driver. To make matters even worse, if the race is on a clockwise circuit, the muscles on the right side of the neck will take more of a hammering than those on the left.

Upper body strength is also important when it comes to the physical effort of driving a race or rally car. The simple fact is that weak muscles will quickly tire and prevent a driver from maintaining peak performance.

Bernie Shrosbree (previously Human Performance Manager at Renault F1) says...
A man off the street who considers himself very fit would only last a few laps of a typical Formula 1 race circuit. The next day he would struggle to even lift his head off the pillow. That's how tough the G-forces are on your neck.

How strong do you need to be for racing?

As with any of the aspects of fitness examined in this book, you know if you are not operating at a sufficiently high level when fatigue of some sort limits your performance. In the case of strength, this will emerge as tired, tight, and sore muscles during or immediately after competition. The effect of these tired muscles will be to make you uncomfortable, reduce concentration levels, and impair your ability to move and react with speed and precision. Therefore, once you have identified the areas of weakness, a programme that emphasises working those particular muscle groups, whilst not ignoring all-round conditioning, is the best plan. The exercises in this chapter form the basis of a balanced strength workout covering the main muscle groups needed for competitive driving.

OPPOSITE: Jarno Trulli working his upper body during driver-training in Kenya before the 2002 season. *(Renault F1)*

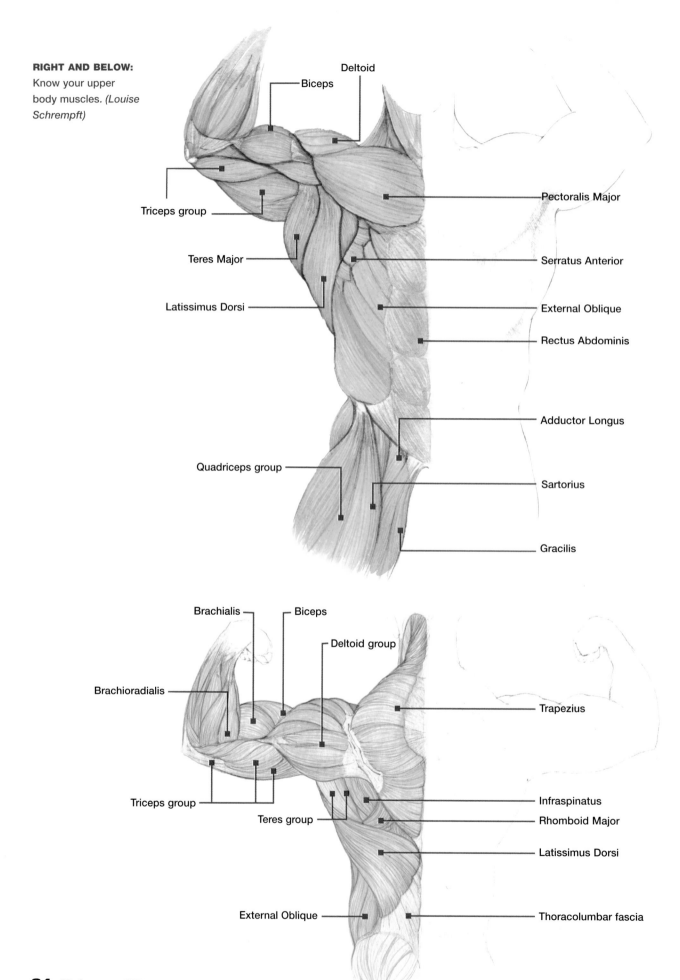

RIGHT AND BELOW:
Know your upper
body muscles. *(Louise
Schrempft)*

Deltoid

Biceps

Triceps group

Teres Major

Latissimus Dorsi

Quadriceps group

Pectoralis Major

Serratus Anterior

External Oblique

Rectus Abdominis

Adductor Longus

Sartorius

Gracilis

Brachialis

Biceps

Deltoid group

Brachioradialis

Trapezius

Triceps group

Teres group

Infraspinatus

Rhomboid Major

Latissimus Dorsi

External Oblique

Thoracolumbar fascia

As well as enhancing performance, racers also need to be strong to contend with the monumental levels of force that the body can be subjected to during a crash. It almost goes without saying that a robust physique, particularly in the trunk or core area, will withstand more punishment than a weak one – and this will lead to quicker recovery rates and fewer injuries should the worst happen. Think of your resistance plan as an insurance policy against injury and time out of the car, then the time you dedicate to it will seem like a wise investment.

Chris Pfeiffer (2007 Indoor Streetbike Freestyle World Champion) recognises the importance of strength training…
Strength training never was my passion but the older I get the more important it is to keep my muscular balance. I now have no more back pain, thanks to the appropriate strength training.

Knowing the lingo

For benefit, muscles must be exposed to overload. They then get bigger and stronger, a process known as hypertrophy. The number of times you perform an exercise without stopping is known as the repetitions, or 'reps' as some like to call them. Although there is no optimum number of repetitions, higher numbers (between 10 and 30) are preferable for racers, as this type of work is good for building strength endurance without creating large muscle bulk. Starting with a weight or level of resistance that allows around ten reps, then building up the number that can be completed, is a safer way of progressing resistance work at first, rather than simply increasing the load lifted.

A set is a collective term for a number of repetitions. Again, many recommend a start of just one or two sets, with a progressive build-up to three or even four as strength develops.

Resistance is the load that you are working against. It may simply be in weight measures such as kilograms or a scale, for example one to ten.

Progressive muscular resistance training is when you choose a number of repetitions at a given weight and gradually increase the amount of reps done over time. Once a high level of reps are attainable (i.e. 20-30, depending on the exercise) increasing the weight very slightly keeps the overload applied to stimulate further improvements.

BELOW: A member of the public, even if very fit, would only last a few laps of a typical F1 race. *(GEPA Pictures/ Red Bull Photofiles)*

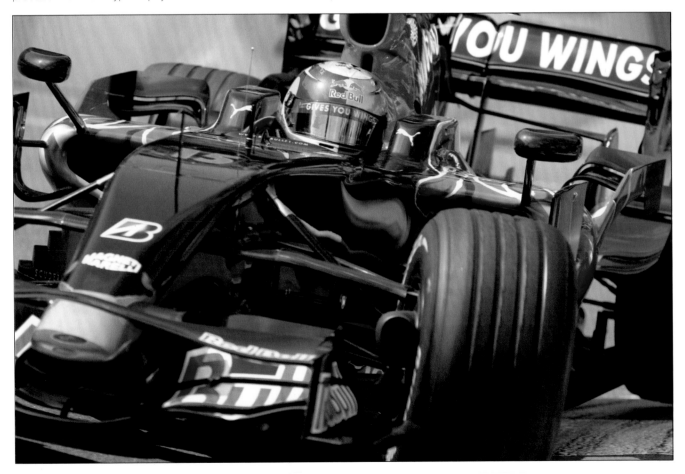

How much to do

When starting a strength training programme, decide what you want to achieve. Chart your performance in a diary and regularly measure your muscles on a three-week basis by performing a test set. Try to workout at least three to five times a week as this has been shown to be most effective. A good start is 1 or 2 sets of 10 repetitions every other day. As a general rule, a lower number of repetitions at higher loads builds strength. A higher number of repetitions at lower loads leads to strength endurance. For racers, strength endurance is generally a higher priority – however, some pure strength work with slightly lower reps is beneficial as general conditioning improves.

Remember that working with heavy weights can be dangerous. Safety is always a priority. Be sensible and start with low weights, and make sure that you rest for about a minute between sets, and at least two days between particularly heavy workouts, to allow your muscles to recover. Try to alternate muscle groups so the same muscles are not always stressed. Interspersing days of strength-training with days of aerobic work (see Chapter 3) is a sensible way to begin training and reduce the chance of excessive muscle soreness.

Super Sport lap record holder at TT Assen, Netherlands, Iain McPherson recognises that upper body strength is important for his sport. But, he knows that a too bulky and muscular body can also be a hindrance. He prefers to do resistance work and concentrates largely on press-ups and pull-ups.

Session planning

All strength-training exercises should be performed after a good warm-up. Suitable warm-up activities include rowing, jogging, cycling, or even doing controlled body weight exercises. The main criteria are that body and muscle temperature are elevated to help avoid tears and strains (see Chapter 2). For ideas on flexibility and mobilisation work that can be incorporated into the warm-up, see Chapter 5. Although stretching before training is generally considered unnecessary, it may be useful if you have particular flexibility issues that would otherwise limit your range of motion.

A range of between six and ten exercises is usually the optimum number for one session, and trying not to focus exclusively on one body part is certainly best when starting out. Use the mirrors in the gym, or a knowledgeable training partner, to help ensure that you maintain excellent technique when strength training, as injury is often the penalty for not doing so.

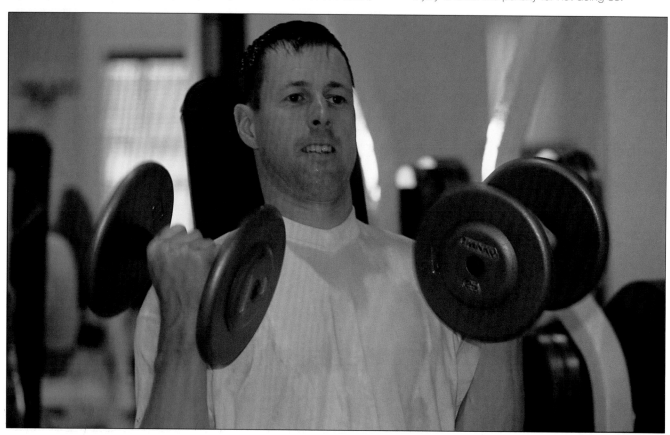

Suggested exercises for racing drivers

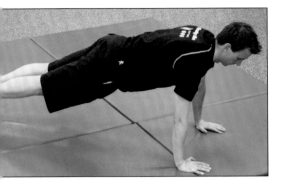

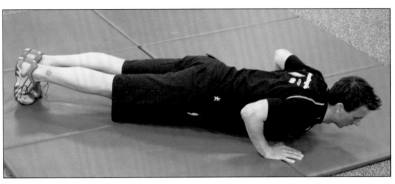

1 Press-ups – three variations (standard on knees and full press-ups, feet on gym ball and hands on bars or dumbbells)

Press-ups are the classic upper body strengthening exercise. They are also very often performed badly, so paying attention to good technique is very important. Proper technique involves maintaining a straight line from knee to hip to shoulder throughout the movement (i.e. no arching of the back or sagging from the hips). Try to make sure you inhale as you lower the chest towards the floor and exhale as you press up. Imagine that you are being pulled up from the hips to maintain the flat position throughout. Primarily they work the pectorals, anterior deltoids and triceps, but because of the high level of static work done by the trunk they are an excellent and underrated exercise for abs and lower back too.

They can be performed with knees down for women (poor technique or lack of strength when performing full press-ups can place a strain on the uterus) or anyone lacking the strength in the trunk to complete the full exercise.

An interesting variation for motor racers is using press-ups bars and a Swiss ball to increase the specificity of the hand and wrist position, and to place even more stress on the core area.

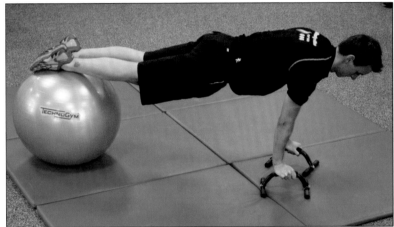

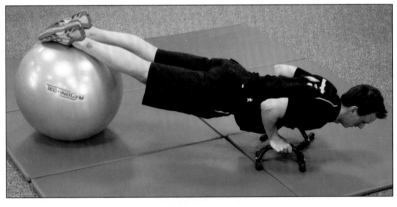

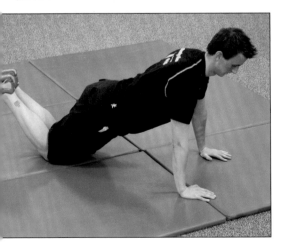

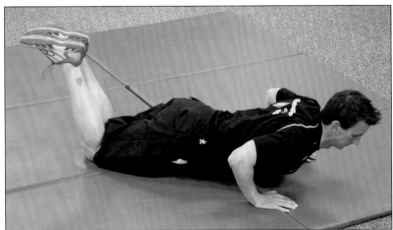

RIGHT AND BELOW:
Chin-ups and chest heaves. Both these develop core strength as well as the upper body. *(Dave Blow, myeyefor)*

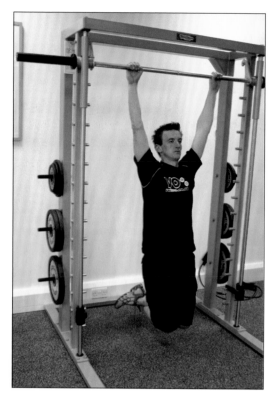

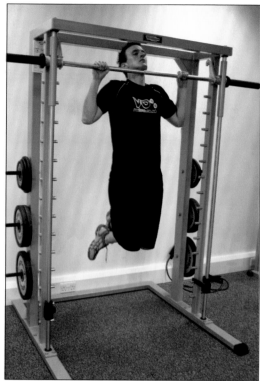

2 Chin-ups and chest heaves

These exercises target latissimus dorsi, posterior deltoids, lower trapezius, and biceps, and they improve grip strength – all good points for drivers. Chin-ups are a very tough exercise as you have to pull your entire bodyweight vertically, so either chest heaves or a machine that uses a counterweight are the best place to start from scratch.

As shown, chest heaves are done under a low bar with your feet on the floor. The higher the bar, the easier the exercise becomes. The key is to maintain tension in the core area so as not to sag down or flick the hips as you raise and lower the body. Simply hanging off the bar is excellent to develop grip strength when starting out, if you cannot complete many reps.

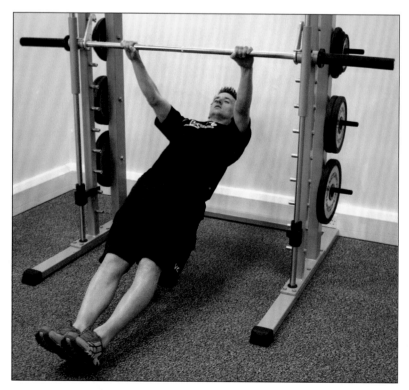

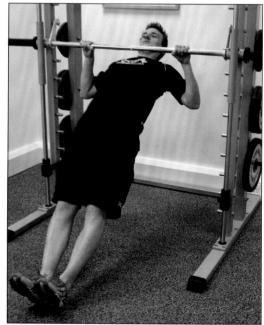

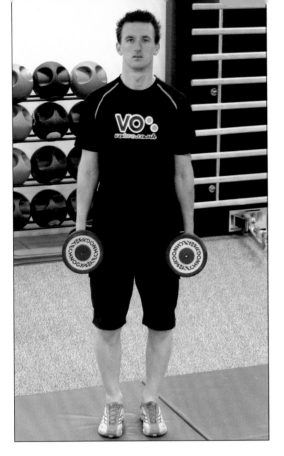

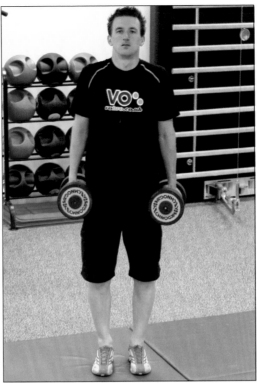

LEFT: Shoulder shrugs. It is important to let the weights down in a controlled manner rather than simply letting them drop. (Dave Blow, myeyefor)

3 Shoulder shrugs

These exercises are good for pose value in the gym, as you get to hold some pretty big dumbbells! Very simply, you hold the weights by your sides and shrug the shoulders upwards to work upper trapezius and improve grip strength. Keep your chin tucked in and remember to control the weights on the way down rather than simply letting them drop. This helps maintain the correct length of your arms too!

4 Lateral raise

Working the deltoids and rotator cuff muscles (that are critical for shoulder stability), lateral

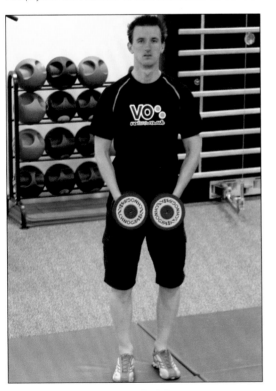

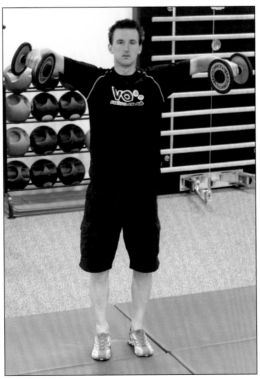

LEFT: Try to perform the lateral raises as smoothly as possible to prevent damage to the delicate rotator cuff muscles. (Dave Blow, myeyefor)

RIGHT AND BELOW:
The reverse cable
cross-over with the
ideal body positioning.
(Dave Blow, myeyefor)

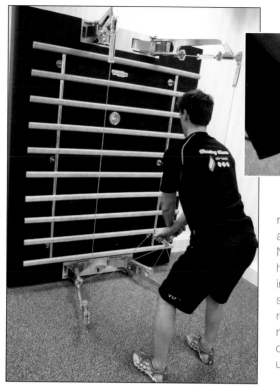

raises should be performed in a smooth
and controlled way throughout the motion.
Note the start point of the exercise, with
hands in front of the body (this helps to avoid
impingement injuries in the shoulder) and arms
subtly flexed at the elbow. Keep the weight
relatively light on these and perform a high
number of reps. Rotator cuff muscles can be
quite delicate, and swinging big iron around is
unnecessarily risky.

5 Reverse cable cross-over

Very rarely performed, this is an excellent
postural exercise for drivers, as it targets the
muscles of the upper back – rhomboids,
deltoids, and upper trapezius. The lower
trunk area also gets used heavily in stabilising
the position. As ever, smooth movements
are essential to avoid jerking the back. Be
modest in the selection of weight as the
upper back muscles are relatively small and
weak compared with those of the chest and
arms, aiming for high reps rather than high
resistance. Check that you are bending from
the hips rather than rounding the shoulders, a
staggered stance with one leg slightly in front
of the other often helps this.

6 Seated row

This exercise brings in the muscles of the
lower back and is performed in a seated
position not too dissimilar to that in the car.
The main muscles used are lumbar erector
spinae and biceps, with grip strength once
more being tested. Ensure that you lean
forward from the hips (think about sitting tall)
so that you are not bending over too much
and loading the lumbar discs. Relatively slow
and controlled movements in and out are best,
and if you find that you are suffering pins and
needles in your feet, try bending the knees
slightly to relieve the stretch on the sciatic
nerve.

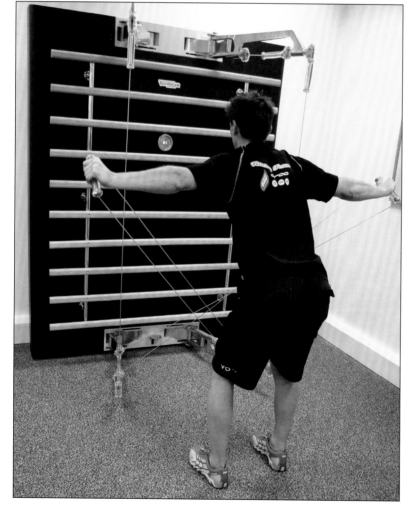

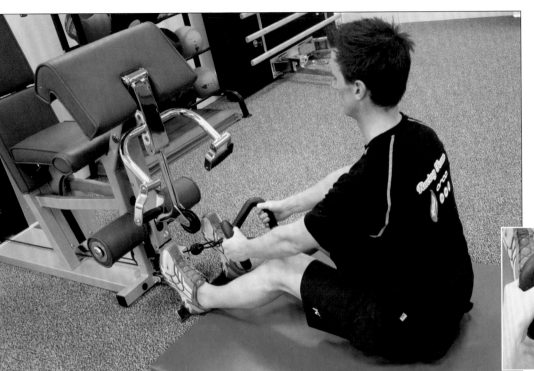

LEFT AND BELOW:
The seated row
simulates the driving
position and works on
the erector spinae and
biceps muscles. *(Dave
Blow, myeyefor)*

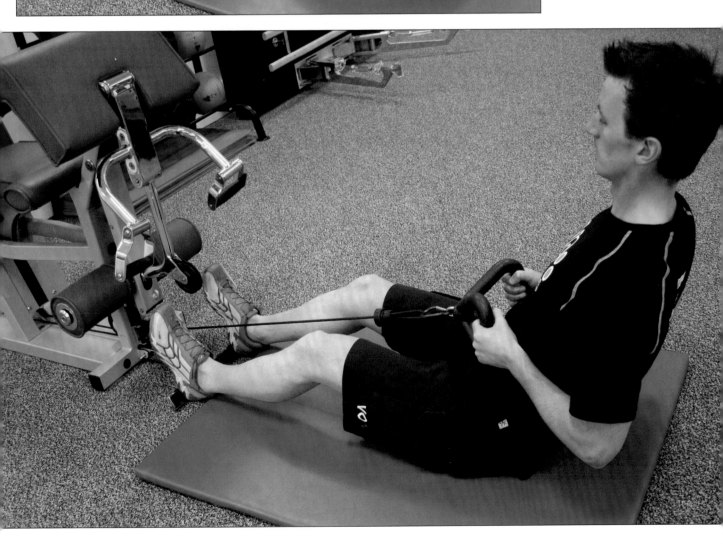

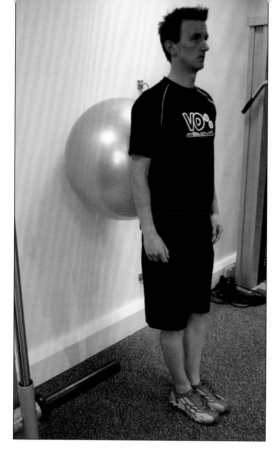

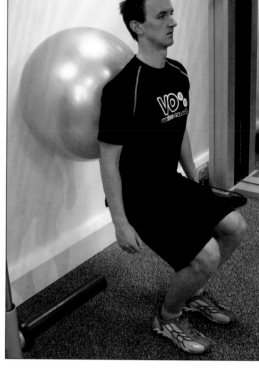

7 Ball squats

Working the quadriceps, gluteals, and trunk, ball
squats are a safe alternative to squatting with a
heavy bar. Lean into the ball with it supporting your
lower back. As you squat down keep your heels
on the floor and push up through them as you get
to about 90 degrees. Start with body weight only,
and progress to holding dumbbells as you get
stronger. Do not let your backside slip backwards

under the ball as you lower down. Maintain tension
in your trunk to keep your back straight and stop
this from occurring. Watch that you don't hold your
breath while doing this.

8 Heel raise

As above, but keeping your leg straight and going
up on tip toes (one leg at a time). This works the
calf muscles at the back of the lower leg.

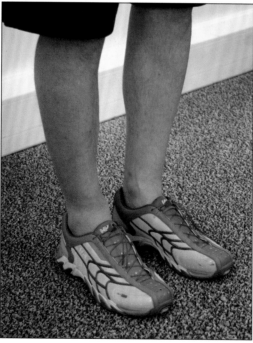

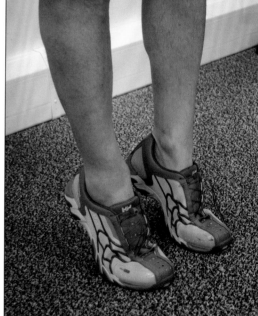

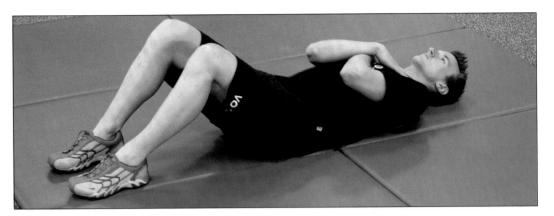

LEFT AND BELOW:
Abdominal crunches are well recognised for their versatility and effectiveness. Performed with a Swiss ball, they offer even more benefits. *(Dave Blow, myeyefor)*

9 Crunches

These abdominal or 'ab' exercises can be performed on the floor or on a Swiss ball to add instability and work the trunk more dynamically. Key points are: ensure that you are breathing correctly and deeply throughout (inhale as you lower, exhale as you raise up) and keep your neck relaxed and spine in a straight line (holding a tennis ball under your chin helps with this at first).

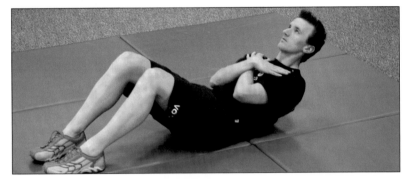

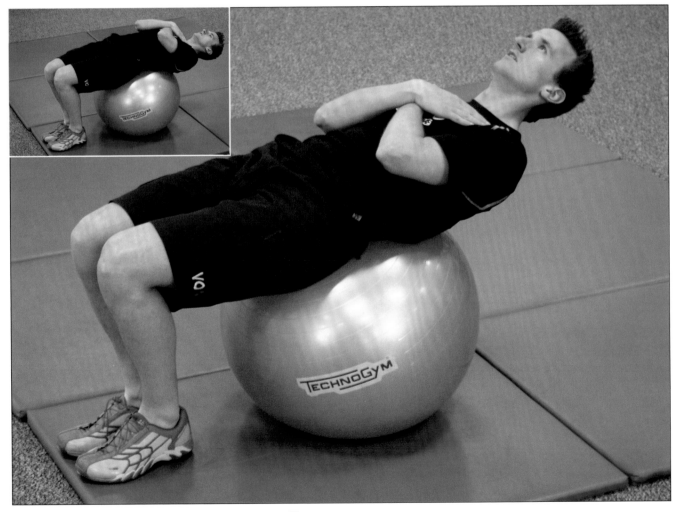

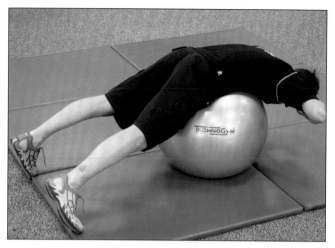

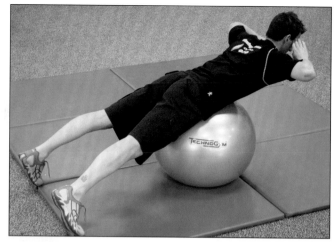

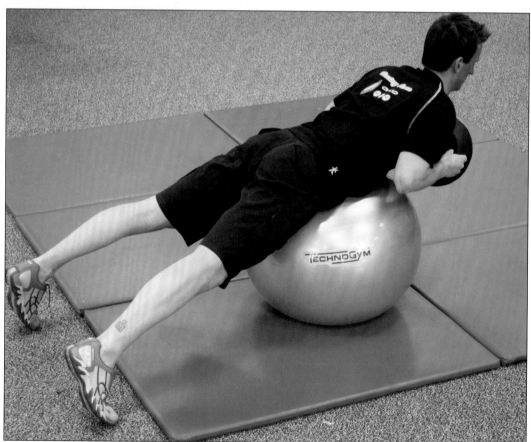

10 Back extensions

Lying on your front with the ball supporting your pelvis, lift your upper body upwards until your back is extended. Control the movement both on the way up and down. There is no particular reason why you cannot hyperextend the back as long as it is done smoothly and steadily. Placing your feet against a wall helps to keep them on the ground, and holding a weight to your chest increases the resistance of the exercise. Be sure to start with bodyweight only first, and be conservative in the way you introduce weight to this movement. Back

extensions work the muscle lumbar erector spinae primarily, and are an excellent complement to crunches and other abdominal work to maintain a good ratio of strength in the stomach and lower back areas.

Other exercises relevant to driving

Swiss ball work

A Swiss ball is a giant rubber inflatable sphere used to provide an unstable platform for exercising

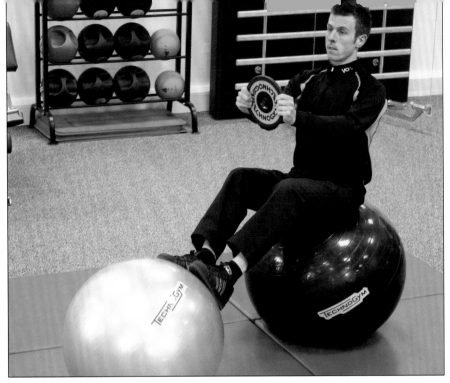
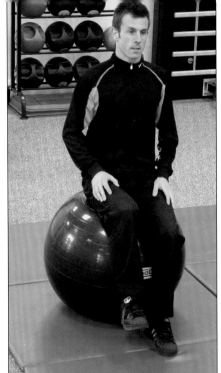
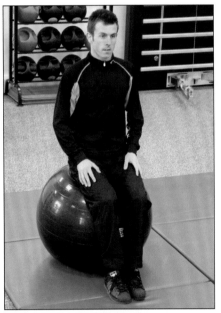
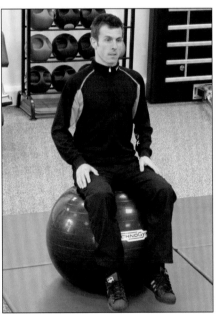
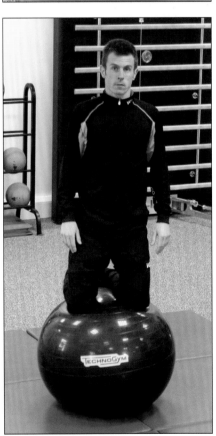
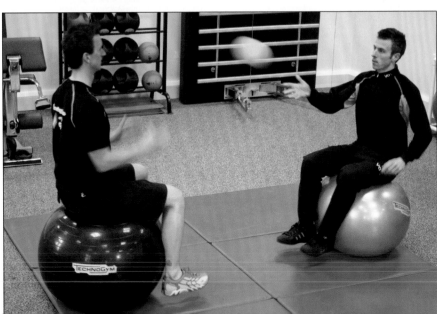

THIS PAGE: The Swiss ball is easily adapted to motorsport. While seated on the ball, with either one foot or both feet off the ground, the body core is activated. As core body strength and balance improves, try kneeling or even passing a ball to someone else with both feet off the ground. *(Dave Blow, myeyefor)*

Example Swiss Ball exercises for drivers

Seated position. You can begin the process of activating the core muscle groups by simply sitting on the ball. Begin with feet down, then one foot up and eventually with both feet up. Once you have mastered this you can bring in other exercises such as throwing and catching drills, shoulder and arm raises or progressions to kneeling and standing (!) to further develop the trunk.

Driving position stability. When you have mastered the feet-up seated position, to make it even more specific to the driving position you can introduce a second ball to rest your feet on. Start with a small football or medicine ball and try to maintain stability in the trunk whilst you perform upper body movements such as steering wheel rotations or wrist exercises as shown.

Neck specific exercises. One of the constant problems for motor racers is how to condition the neck for the high G forces associated with fast single-seater racing. For this one you need a partner to help you. Sit on the ball with your feet close together and on the floor. Get your partner to place their hand on your forehead and apply a moderate resistance. You have to match that resistance statically with your neck muscles whilst maintaining good posture, and hold it for two or three seconds. Without fully releasing the tension, your helper then moves their hand to a different place on your head and you continue to statically resist their pressure at a different angle. Repeat the process in various positions to work the neck from all angles. You will notice that all of the trunk muscles are brought into play on this too. Simply build up the amount of time you can hold the resistance for, and maybe in time try it with one foot off the ground as you become stronger and more skilled.

BELOW: With aggressive strength training, Stuntriding Indoor World Champion Chris Pfeiffer can now withstand such landings that would have otherwise affected his back. *(rutgerpauw. com/Red Bull Photofiles)*

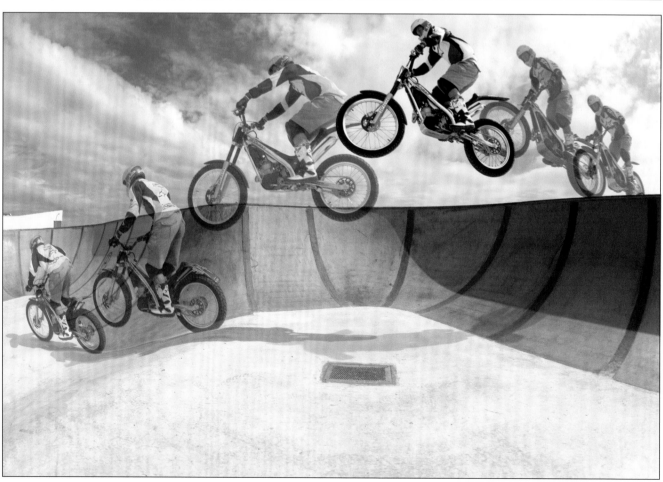

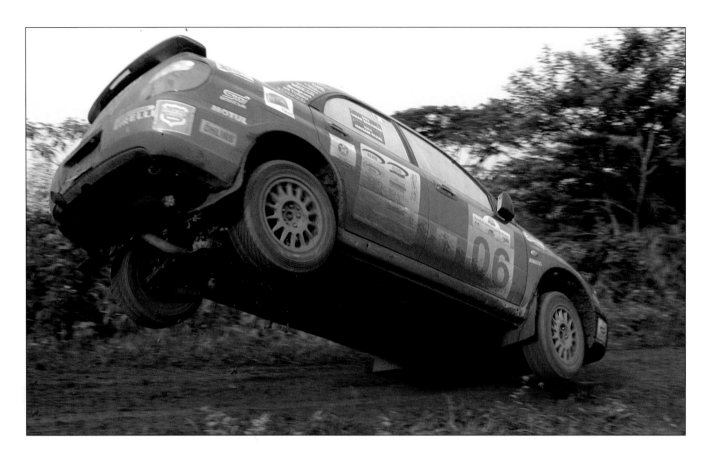

on. There is a growing body of evidence showing that simply sitting on a ball switches on the body's core control muscles (mainly located in the trunk area). By using a ball in your strength-training sessions you help the body to differentiate between muscles used in stabilisation and muscles used for movement whilst driving. This is critical to build core strength up to levels that can help to protect vital organs, the skeleton, and joints, as they can be subjected to extremely high forces in crashes which inevitably occur in motor sport from time to time.

Dr Jonathan Whelan (Chief Medical Officer, Thruxton Race Circuit)...

Speaking as an emergency doctor on race events, it is clear that those competitors who have greater core strength deal easier with their crashes and mishaps. They seem to walk away from the accidents, unlike those who need to develop this essential part of their fitness.

The underlying principle of strength training is that during the session muscles are stressed and mildly damaged in order to stimulate repair and growth during recovery periods afterwards. Naturally, this damage can result in soreness and stiffness which is at its worst when you first begin a resistance programme. A day or two after your first lifting session, expect to feel a little like you have been run over by a bus, but rest assured that before too long your body will adapt and you will recover more readily!

In conclusion, strength training is an essential aspect of conditioning for motorsport. Use this chapter in conjunction with the rest of the book to keep performing at your best for the whole race, and ready to protect yourself if it all goes wrong!

Andy Blow on strength training for drivers...

Any racing driver has a responsibility to prepare themselves to the best of their ability so they are not only strong enough to cope with the physical demands of racing, but also the exceptional forces that the body can be subjected to in an accident.

References

Willardson, J. M. 'Core stability training: applications to sports conditioning programs', *J. Strength Cond. Res.* 2007; 21(3):979-85.

ABOVE: Heavy landings like these can cause considerable injury to the body unless core body strength is worked on. *(Anwar Sidi Images)*

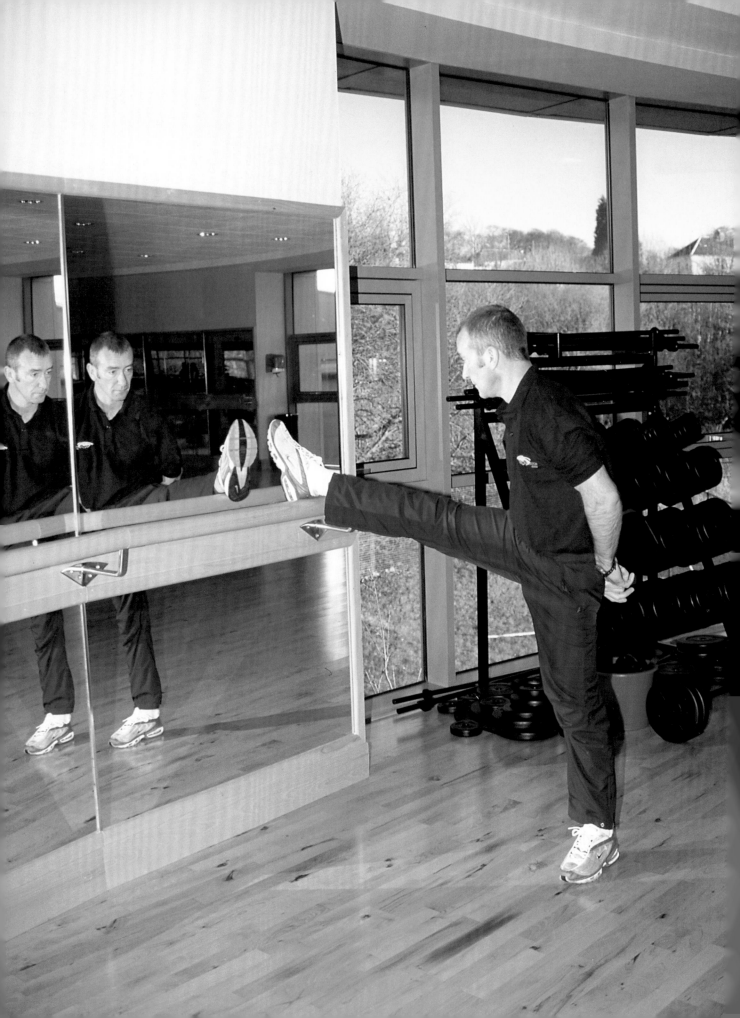

5

Suppleness (or flexibility)

This is the extent to which the structures in the body can be stretched without actually being damaged. The question 'how flexible are you?' is a very subjective one, and the answer depends on a number of factors, such as the position you drive in, what part of the body you are looking at and even the temperature.

If you do not have the necessary flexibility for your driving position you risk early fatigue, injury, poor injury recovery, and of course PAIN. You need to be flexible enough to spend prolonged periods of time in the driving position. You need to be able to make all the necessary movements to drive and maintain awareness of what is going on around you, and still have enough flexibility in reserve in case you are involved in an accident and your body is rapidly pushed beyond the range it normally moves in.

Flexibility training should be carried out in conjunction with strengthening work. As you gain more movement you need to be able to control this. Flexibility that you have little or no control over can be just as harmful as poor flexibility. If you apply the principles discussed in the strengthening chapter to your increased range of motion, this can lead to enhanced performance and prevention of injury.

This chapter should be used as a guide for you to form your own flexibility programme. The exercises for the core should be addressed by all those who are in the car when it is being raced. The peripheral exercises you choose to take from this chapter will depend on the experiences that you yourself have had in the car.

Preparing to stretch

Preparation for stretching should not be neglected. The tissues in your body are much more pliable when they are warm, so make sure that you have warmed up thoroughly prior to stretching. Spend 10 to 15 minutes doing a low intensity warm-up first. Revisit Chapter 2 to check that you are doing this effectively. If you're doing this outdoors or in a drafty gym, make sure you wear the appropriate clothing to stay warm and protect yourself from the elements. How much time you spend stretching will depend on how much work your flexibility needs and how many areas of your body need attention. Try to work in sets of three to five, and adjust depending on your own experiences. Time spent stretching should be anywhere from 20 minutes to an hour each day. You need to do enough to cover all the parts of the body that need attention, but not so much that you lose interest. Remember that you don't need to address every body part in every session, so break up the sessions.

What should I stretch?

Motorsport driving places stresses on particular parts of the body. Your stretching programme should be tailored not only on areas of the body that are commonly working hard in motor racing, but also on areas that you find are specifically loaded when YOU drive. Ask yourself some basic questions to begin with:

■ Are there any aspects of my driving position that cause pain?
■ Do I have the joint range or muscle length to

OPPOSITE: Jim Moodie, seven-times winner of the Isle of Man TT, keeps supple by exercising in the gym. *(Mike Gibbon, MVG Photographic)*

do all the necessary movements while I am in that position?

■ Are there any areas of my body which seem to be fatiguing unusually early?

■ Can I look far enough round to stay aware of what is going on around me?

Answering yourself these questions should help you to tailor your own flexibility programme.

Stretching to relieve and prevent pain

So, how do you go about increasing your own flexibility? You've worked out which areas are hurting, but now you need to know which tight structures are actually causing the pain. The type of pain you get and the behaviour of that pain can be a good indicator. A deep aching pain that starts locally but then spreads out can implicate a restriction in joint and/or ligament movement. Watch out for a sharp pain as you get into the driving position as this may indicate an injury that needs the attention of a health professional. Lack of muscle and/or tendon length can present as rapid fatigue in the driving position, a general tight feeling in the limb and an inability to use the affected limb to carry out tasks when in the driving position. If you have a problem with muscle length you will often find these movements are easy when you are not in the driving position.

Perhaps the most painful restriction is the lack of nerve length or movement. Often termed as poor neural dynamics, or neuropathodynamics, by health professionals, this usually presents as a sharp, burning pain. The driver may often find that over time they develop a pins-and-needles or even a numbing sensation. Sustained or frequent stressing of the nerves in this way can lead to neural irritation, which leads to a toothache-type pain and persistent burning, pins-and-needles or numbness.

Preventing pain and increasing movement

Prevention is certainly better than cure. It's important to keep all structures flexible to prevent problems. These exercises should form part of your daily routine and can be used before and after training and racing. When rallying, they can be used to keep you supple between stages.

For convenience, we will split the exercise into two groups:

■ peripheries – arms and legs
■ core areas – neck, trunk and back.

You may find that you prefer, for example, to address the upper body then the lower body. Either way, try to establish a routine that works for you and one you can remember without frequent reference to a list of exercises. This will help you to maintain your flexibility programme.

The periphery
When stretching out your arms and legs, you need to mobilise the joints and ligaments, muscles and tendons, and your nerves.

Arms
Joints
The old cliché 'Use it or lose it' certainly applies here. When mobilising your joints, make sure that you move them through their entire range. Shoulder rotations will help to ensure that they do not become too restricted from the relatively restricted position they can be placed in when you're driving.

Muscles and tendons
These should be stretched in the positions that you are going to be using them in. Active and dynamic stretches have been found in the most up-to-date research to be more effective for increasing movement and preventing injury than the conventional static passive stretches currently used by many sportsmen and women. The stretches should be done slowly and rhythmically and do not really need to be held. Stretching the arm muscles together rather than separately will help to keep the exercises functional to how you are going to be using your arms.

To stretch out the front of the arm and shoulder, reach the arm back and slowly straighten the elbow. Keep the fist loosely clenched and don't pull the wrist back. This will help to prevent the nerves being overstressed by this exercise.

To stretch out the back of the arm and shoulder, reach across the body. Hold the elbow with the other hand and gently pull back against it.

To stretch out the wrist muscles, gently pull back the wrist from the palm and slowly extend the elbow. Do this again, but this time pull back from the fingers. Take care not to allow this to bring on pins-and-needles, numbness, burning or sharp pain.

'Tennis elbow', or lateral epicondylitis, is a pain in the elbow frequently encountered by drivers and can come about as a result of prolonged hard gripping of the steering wheel. It

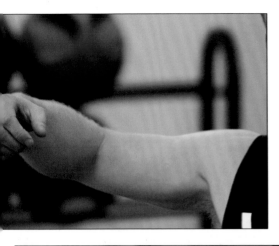
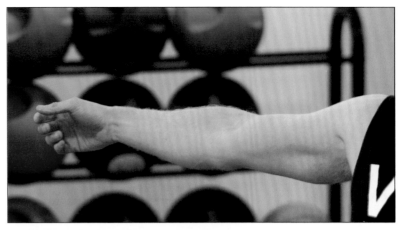

ABOVE LEFT AND RIGHT: These images illustrate how the pectoral muscles and arm can be stretched easily. *(Dave Blow, myeyefor)*

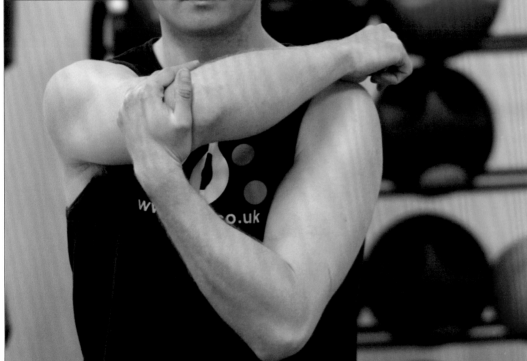

LEFT: The back of the arm and shoulder is stretched. *(Dave Blow, myeyefor)*

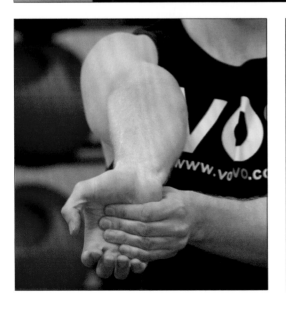
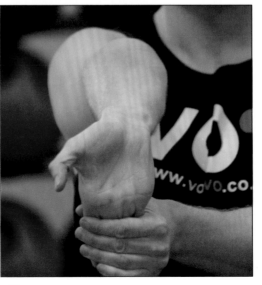

FAR LEFT AND LEFT: Make sure that there is no numbness or tingling when you undertake this exercise that stretches the flexors group. *(Dave Blow, myeyefor)*

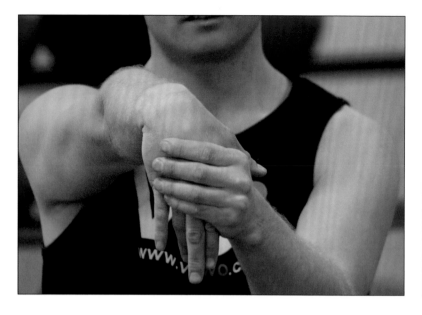

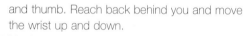

is characterised by a localised pain on the outside, made worse by gripping. To prevent this, pull the wrist down and extend the elbow.

Nerves

When mobilising the nerves, it is important to remember that we are not trying to stretch them. We are just trying to improve how smoothly they move. These exercises may help if you suffer from burning or pins-and-needles when driving. The exercises should elicit a very gentle stretching sensation and must not be painful. They should be done slowly and rhythmically without being held in one position. The three main nerves to focus on in the arm are the ulnar nerve, median nerve, and radial nerve.

- Radial nerve. Restriction here can lead to the neural symptoms around the back of the arm

and thumb. Reach back behind you and move the wrist up and down.
- Median nerve. Restriction at the level of the wrist may lead to a condition known as Carpal Tunnel Syndrome. This manifests itself as pins-and-needles around the palm area, and loss of grip strength. Put yourself into the driving position and straighten your elbow out in front of you while drawing the wrist back.
- Ulnar nerve. Restriction is typically at the level of the elbow, or if the upper arm has been forcibly stretched back causing traction on the nerve as it exits under the armpit. The symptoms are usually pins-and-needles in the little finger and ring finger with associated weakness. Lift your arm out to the side, elbow bent and wrist facing upwards. Circle the hand around as if brushing the hair on the outside of the head backwards.

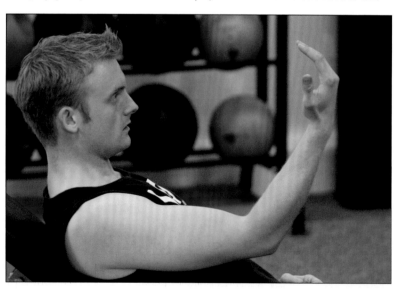

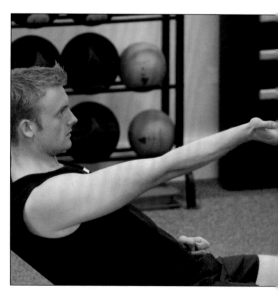

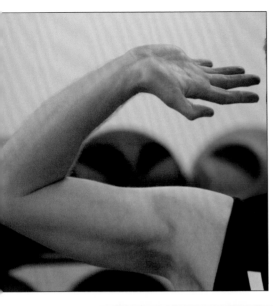

Legs
Joints and ligaments

The joints in the legs of motor sport drivers should not require any specific attention beyond frequently circling the ankles round while in the pit lane or between stages.

Muscles and tendons

Restriction in the hamstrings at the back to the thigh can lead to cramping in this area, and lower back pain while driving. Research shows that you cannot physically increase the length of the hamstrings. You can, however, retrain them to play out with greater ease. Lie on your back and bend the hip up to about 90 degrees. Increase the arch in your back and then straighten the knee. Once the knee is straightened as far as you are able, slowly lower the leg and begin again.

FAR LEFT: The ulnar nerve is usually compressed at the level of the elbow and can be stretched gently using this exercise. *(Dave Blow, myeyefor)*

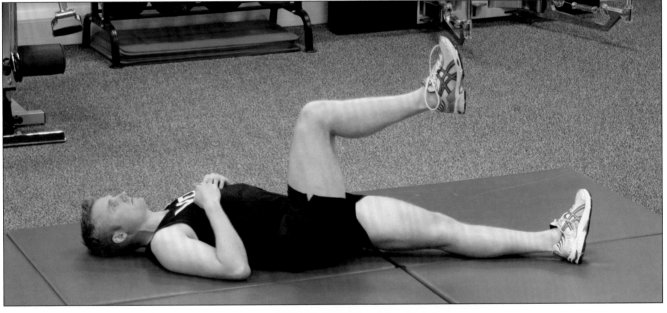

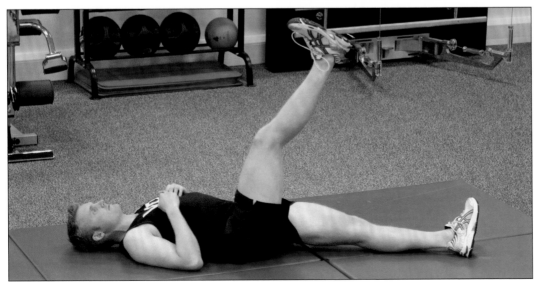

ABOVE AND LEFT: Tight hamstrings can cause lower back pain with driving. This exercise helps loosen the muscles. *(Dave Blow, myeyefor)*

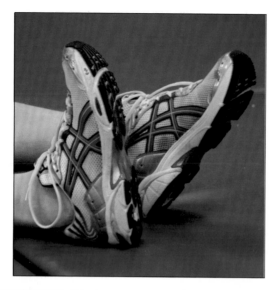

RIGHT: Similarly, tight calf muscles can restrict movement from pedal to pedal. (Dave Blow, myeyefor)

BELOW: Sitting back stretches the front of your ankle. (Dave Blow, myeyefor)

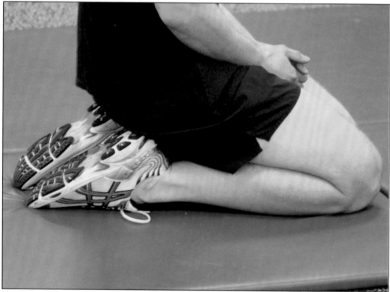

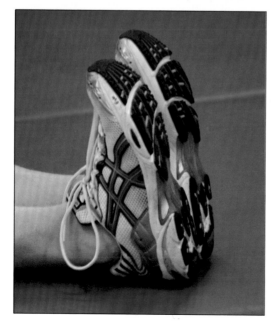

RIGHT: Stretching the sciatic nerve – a common cause of leg pain. (Dave Blow, myeyefor)

Once you have got the hang of this try doing it in your driving position.

Tight calves can lead to cramp and a difficulty moving the feet rapidly from one pedal to another. To stretch them out, sit in your driving position and pull your foot up towards you from the ankle so that you feel a pulling in the back of the calf. If you find that your foot tends to cramp up, then pull back your big toe while doing this.

If you find it difficult to point your toes enough, then stretch back the muscles that cross the front of the ankle.

A tight feeling in the front of the hips as you get out of the car can indicate that you have tight hip flexors. Place the leg you are going to stretch behind you with the knee straight. Lunge down until you feel a stretch at the front of the hip, and then gently release the stretch. Bending the knee of the leg you are stretching will give you a stretch slightly further down the thigh.

Nerves

The main nerve that causes problems in drivers is the sciatic nerve. This runs down the back of the leg. A restriction here can lead to pain along the back of the leg down to the ankle, pins-and-needles or numbness in the foot, and in extreme cases an inability to hold the foot up or prevent the knee flicking back. Persistent problems here should not be ignored and you should seek the advice of a medical professional. To keep the sciatic nerve mobile. sit up with your legs out in front of you and gently pull your ankles backwards and forwards.

The Core

This is an area that all drivers and co-drivers should work on. Its importance is universally stressed in all forms of motorsport. Unless stated otherwise, the exercises here are predominantly joint mobilisations, and so the amount of time they are held for is not particularly important. The exercises should be performed smoothly and, initially, slowly. The speed of the exercise should be gradually increased to roughly mimic the speeds at which your body is moving when you drive.

Let's start with the neck (cervical spine). A common source of pain and restricted joint movement in driving is the adoption of a protracted chin posture. In this position the upper trunk (thoracic) and neck joints are effectively locked out. This is painful as all of the joints are held at their end of range for long periods of time. Try pulling your finger back as far as it can go and it very quickly starts to hurt. You may be placing

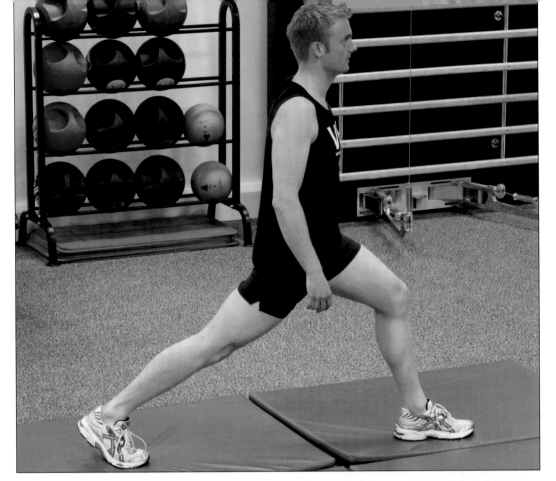

LEFT: Keeping the back leg straight stretches the iliopsoas muscle in front of the hip. *(Dave Blow, myeyefor)*

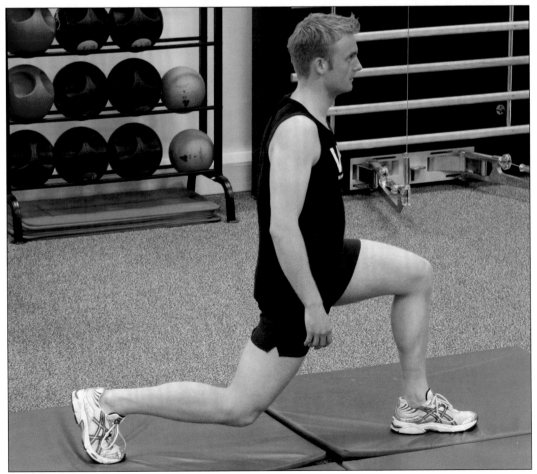

LEFT: Bending the knee of the back leg stretches the rectus femoris muscle. *(Dave Blow, myeyefor)*

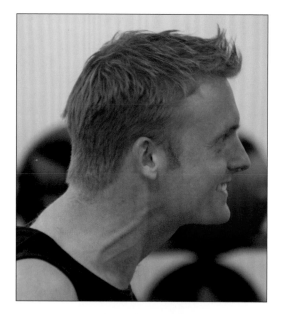

RIGHT: The protracted neck – this is the position NOT to adopt in motorsport. *(Dave Blow, myeyefor)*

RIGHT AND FAR RIGHT: Gentle neck retraction and extension help mobilise the cervical spine which is often subjected to several G-forces during cornering. *(Dave Blow, myeyefor)*

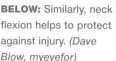

BELOW: Similarly, neck flexion helps to protect against injury. *(Dave Blow, myeyefor)*

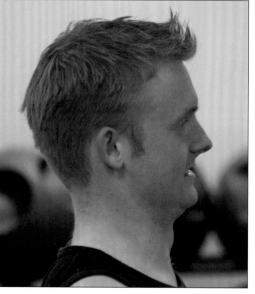

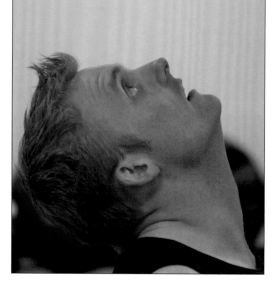

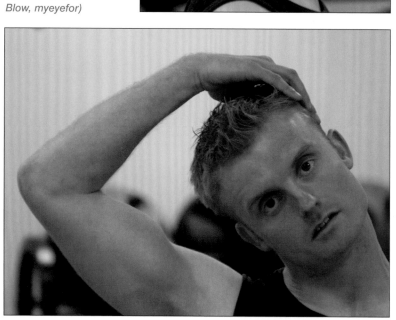

your neck joints in this position for hours at a time. In this position you will also severely restrict the amount of movement that your neck is capable of.

Neck retractions and extensions will help to relieve pain related to this position. Gentle side stretches will help to increase the flexibility of the neck during side-on impacts. This should be done with care to protect the nerves and should certainly not elicit any sharp pain, burning or pins-and-needles.

The upper trunk (thoracic spine) is the part of your spine that the ribs attach to. This is relatively still during motor racing. The driving position tends to lead to the trunk bending forward. The accompanying rounded shoulder position can lead to reduced lung capacity and even chest pain. To counteract this, you should work at extending and rotating the trunk and stretching out the front

of the shoulders. As you hold this stretch, gently try to pull the arm forward as if trying to pull the doorway or training partner towards you. The stretch does not need to be held for any longer than five seconds.

The lower back (lumbar spine) is the part of the spine that normally curves inward as you stand. Inflexibility in this area can lead to back pain and the sensation of tight hamstrings. This curved shape of the spine is your body's natural shock absorber. Maintain this as much as possible and you will be able to absorb more impact from an accident without sustaining an injury. Even with adequate lumbar support, this curve is often reduced or even lost in the driving position. You need to stretch the back in the opposite direction to which it is fixed in when you drive.

It is important that your back has the ability to

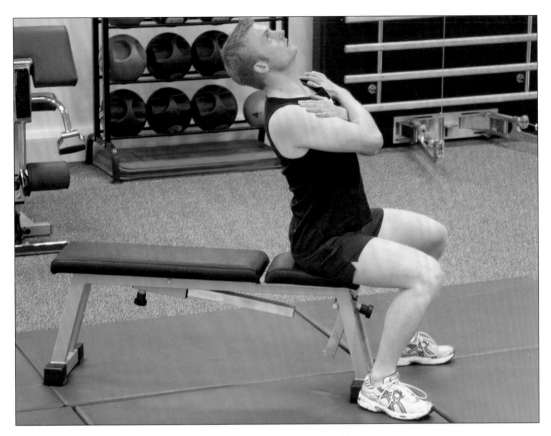

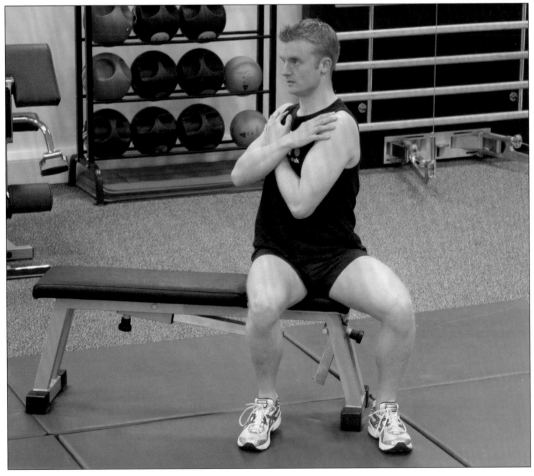

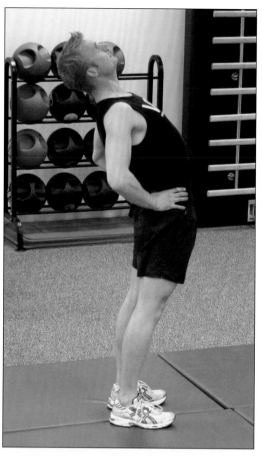

bend forward so that it can tolerate this position
when you're driving. Back flexion exercises should
be incorporated to your back exercises. This is
done by kneeling back on all fours, sitting back on
your ankles and reaching your hands forwards.

The spine flexibility exercises should be
carried out in conjunction with the core stability
work discussed in Chapter 4. Any new range of
movement you gain should be controllable in order
to be useful.

Summary

Take your time to find a flexibility programme that
suits you. Use this chapter as a guide to form it,
and revisit the chapter regularly to modify your
regime as your situation and/or style of driving
changes. Always be aware of the need to consult
a health professional if problems persist or you
think you may have sustained an injury.

Andy Blow on flexibility work...

*Red Bull F1 driver Mark Webber takes his
flexibility training extremely seriously. Using
techniques learnt from Australian Olympic
athletes, he has designed his own routines and
even his own stretching equipment to ensure
his range of movement is optimal for the car
he drives.*

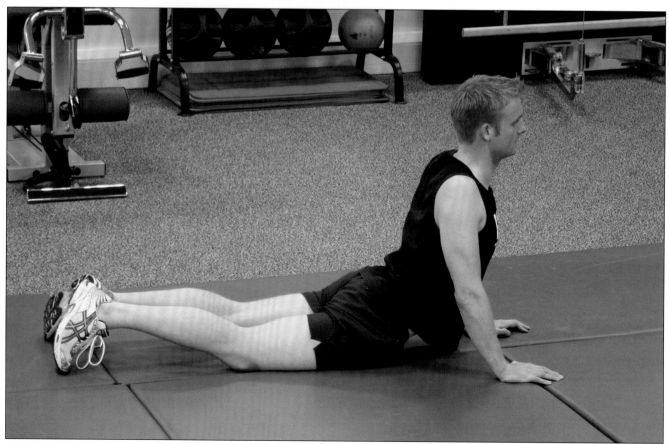

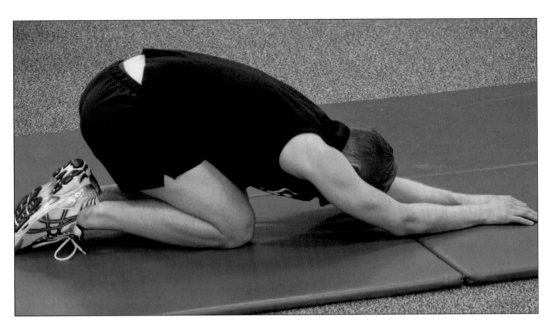

LEFT: An excellent exercise for lower back flexion. (*Dave Blow, myeyefor*)

References

Mahieu, N. et al 'Effect of Static and Ballistic Stretching on the Muscle-Tendon Tissue Properties', *Medicine and Science in Sports and Exercise*, 2007; 39(3): 494-501.

McMillian, D. et al 'Dynamic Versus Static-Stretching Warm Up: The Effect on Power and Agility Performance', *Journal of Strength and Conditioning Research*, 2006; 20(3): 492-499.

Stephens, J. et al 'Lengthening the Hamstring Muscles Without Stretching Using "Awareness Through Movement"', *Physical Therapy*, 2006; 86:1641-1650.

BELOW: Modern race cars such as this 911 GT3 RSR, racing at the Nürburgring 24 Hours, can generate considerable G-forces when cornering, putting the body under significant stress and strain.

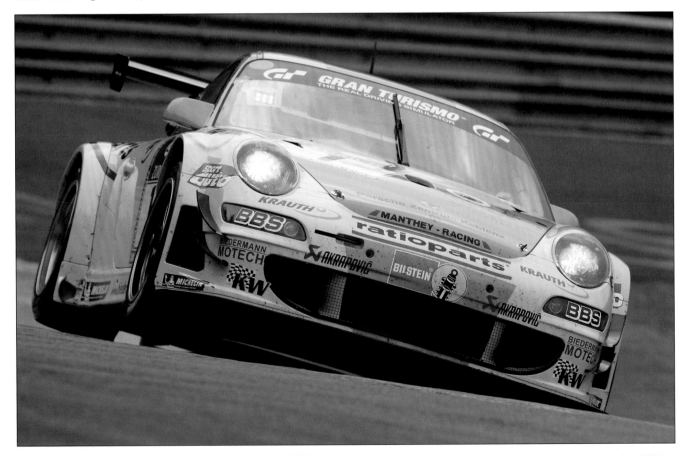

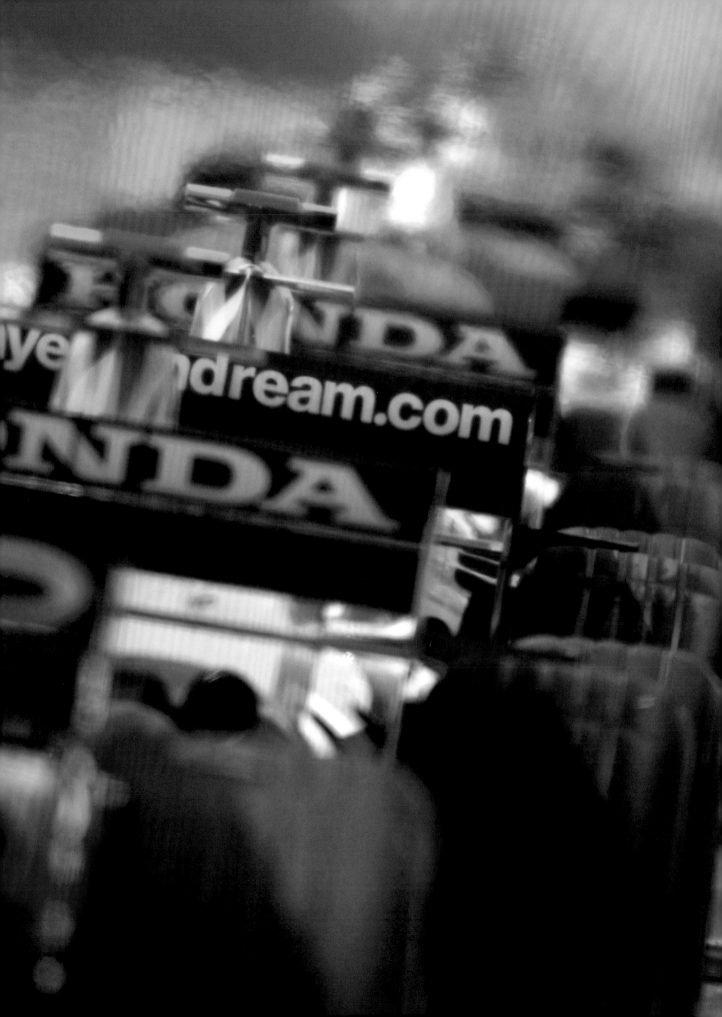

6

Speed

Whilst it is obvious that speed of limb movement is important in many sports, particularly in athletics, its value in motorsport may not be immediately clear. But, think about the need for rapid arm action when trying to keep your car or kart under control, and the benefits become more apparent.

In the context of training and fitness, speed relates to the time taken to perform a task. It incorporates many features of a driver's fitness and is influenced by endurance, strength, mobility, and technique. Speed includes the time taken to react, the reaction or response time (some call it your reflexes), and the time taken to

move your body through the specific task, the movement time. This chapter provides guidance on how to improve your reaction and movement time.

Clearly, a faster reaction time to the lights on the starting grid of a track race will determine who gets to the first corner in the lead. Not uncommonly this also determines who wins the race. However, reaction time is not all about focusing on the start lights and setting off faster than your competitors (cue detection). It is also of importance when the driver has to make a decision, often within a split second, and not uncommonly as a life-saving move. In motorsport,

OPPOSITE: The start of a Formula 1 Grand Prix. Not uncommonly, the race is lost if the driver fails to secure a top position at the first corner.
(MVG Photographic/ Mike Gibbon)

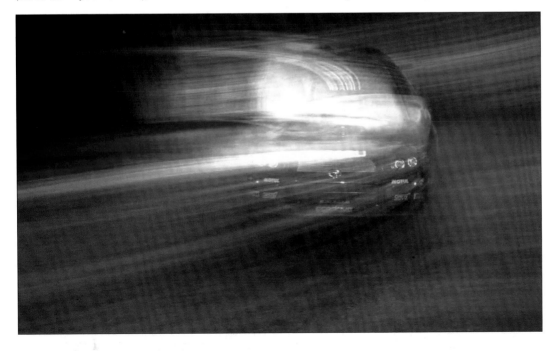

LEFT: Keeping your car on the track calls for quick reactions, particularly when throwing it round twisty rally stages at night, like this WRC Subaru driver.
(MVG Photographic/ Mike Gibbon)

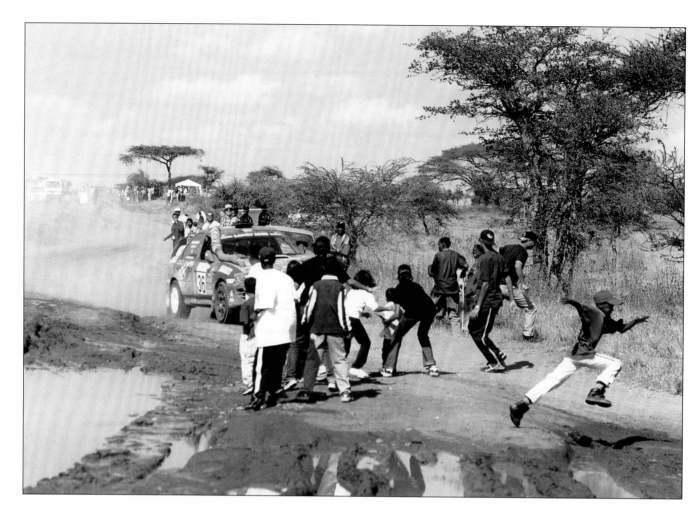

reaction time is a function of both your state of mind (psychology) and your body (physiology). Mentally alert and prepared drivers have a shorter response time, as do those who have been practising. The psychology is discussed later in the book. Other factors that influence reaction times are:

■ Level of anticipation
■ Experience of competitor
■ Number of possible responses available for the situation
■ Time available for the reaction
■ Potential outcome – a life-saving situation will generally provoke a more intense response.

In motorsport, driver response time has also got its safety implications. Your ability to avoid an unexpected rock or an unwary spectator who wanders on to a rally stage is a function of your reaction and movement time.

Bernie Shrosbree feels speed and response time is often underrated in motorsport. In his time as Human Performance Manager at Renault F1, he used the Batak Wall for the drivers. He says:

The Batak system allows the Renault F1 Human Performance Centre to accurately assess a driver's agility and motor response time to a set of random lights. This can be performed under normal or fatigued conditions to simulate the effect of a long race. The system incorporates elements of decision-making into some of the tasks to add a cognitive element to the tests. Tests can last anywhere from 30 seconds to 10 minutes – which can be extremely taxing.

Developing and improving your speed

Just like strength, speed is specific to the sport you compete in. You will find that top drivers are very quick with their hands and feet because they need the quick gear changes and fancy footwork in the car during the race.

It's true that some people are naturally faster than others. This, to some extent, results from their inherited muscle type. Broadly speaking, there are three types of muscle fibre – Types I, IIa and IIb.

Type I fibres (also known as red, or slow-twitch fibres) allow us to perform low-intensity exercises

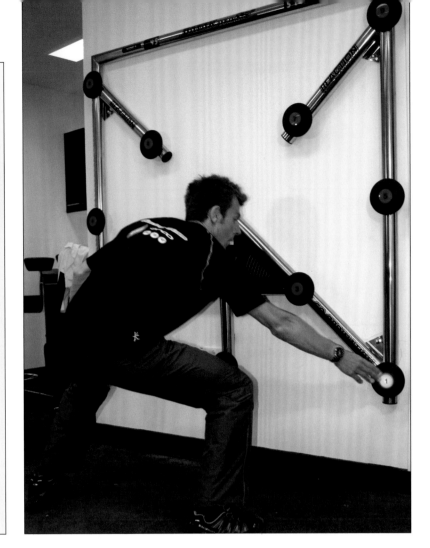

for longer periods, i.e. they have a higher aerobic capacity and therefore fatigue less quickly. Type IIa fibres perform both low and high intensity work in moderate amounts. Type IIb fibres, also known as white or fast-twitch fibres, have the potential to work extremely fast. However, they fatigue more quickly.

Do not despair if you think you are lacking in fast-twitch muscles. The good news is that research has shown that training improves both types, possibly fast-twitch muscles more than slow-twitch.

Speed training is best developed by simulating conditions that you will eventually be competing in. Try to replicate the motions that you expect to make during cornering, braking and so on, and add resistance to the movements. This method of training is well established with top athletes. For example, some sprinters sprint while towing a weight, such as a car tyre behind them or creating drag with a chute to provide resistance. Generally you will build up speed if you make your muscles contract rapidly against a low resistance. Try the following exercises designed to develop faster hands and feet for motorsport.

Faster hands

Boxers need fast hands for their sport. This is achieved using a speed bag which not only improves reaction time but also hand-eye coordination and rhythm. The bag, which is ideally positioned at nose level, also conditions the upper arms and deltoid muscles essential for motorsport drivers.

Internationally renowned speed bag expert Alan Kahn, based in Texas, states…
The drivers of high speed autos have to be in top shape with quickness and immaculate reaction times to handle the speeds they drive at for many hours. Even the slower rides over rough terrain demand top levels of fitness.

If a speed bag is not available then a conventional heavy bag is suitable. Speed drills with this bag involve throwing punches as fast as possible using a minimum of four punches per combination.

Another excellent way to test your reaction time and hand speed, as well as hand-eye coordination, is the commercially available Z-Ball.

ABOVE: The Batak Wall, which measures your reaction time, coordination and balance, was invented by Dr David Nelson. It involves hitting the light as soon as you see it lit. The wall shown in the photograph is used by Porsche Performance Centre drivers. Batak Walls are now commonly used in many sports disciplines. Further information may be obtained on www.batakpro.com. *(Dave Blow, myeyefor)*

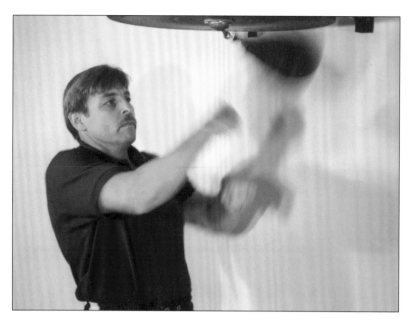

ABOVE: Developing faster hands with the aid of the speed bag, as demonstrated by Alan Kahn – internationally renowned speed bag expert who believes the speed bag helps build upper body strength as well as faster hands with improved hand-eye coordination – all important skills for competitive driving. *(Alan Kahn)*

RIGHT: The SAQ Programme improves multi-directional speed, agility and quickness and overall reaction/ response times. The best way to experience it is to study one of their quick courses and before you know it you will be applying new practical skills and seeing performance across the board reach new heights. Further information may be obtained at www. saqinternational.com *(SAQ International)*

This uniquely designed ball bounces in a random and unpredictable manner and is quite fun and challenging. If played against an opponent it will give you an idea of how you stand. The same can be said for some arcade games. To get even closer to home, some drivers regularly play driving games, such as Colin McRae Rally, on their computers.

Racquet sports, such as squash, table tennis, and badminton are excellent ways to hone your reaction time and hand-eye co-ordination. Carlos Sainz, twice FIA World Rally Champion was also Spanish junior squash champion. Jim Moodie and Alister McRae are squash partners whenever their busy racing calendars allow it.

Faster feet

A simple exercise that requires no equipment is

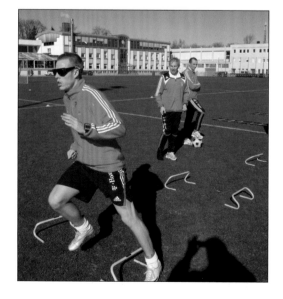

to start jogging on the spot and gradually build up the pace whilst remaining on the same spot. As your speed increases, concentrate on taking controlled steps. They will naturally involve less knee lift, and you may even find it easier to stoop slightly forwards as the speed increases. Another simple drill, used regularly by the armed forces, involves the use of tyres laid flat. The idea is to make your way as fast as possible across the tyres by placing a foot in each tyre. Instead of tyres you can use markers such as items of clothing. For variety, do the exercises whilst facing sideways or even backwards.

One of the most popular methods used by specialist trainers involves the speed-agility ladder measuring 10 yards in length with 18 inch squares. The speed-agility ladder is now readily available to members of the public and is exceptionally easy to use. More details and exercises with the ladder are provided in Chapter 8. Specialist coaches use various other methods for improving foot speed. One drill that develops proprioception (derived from Latin *proprius*, meaning 'one's own', and perception) as well as speed involves the use of a mini-trampoline. Proprioception is the body's unconscious ability to sense what each part is doing – for example, even if you are blindfolded you will know if your leg is extended or not. Not only will you develop proprioception, but the mini-trampoline burns up to 700kcal per hour, develops aerobic endurance, strengthens muscles as well as being a zero-impact exercise. Stepping and bouncing exercises are easy to perform on the mini-trampoline. Drills should take 5-10 seconds initially at a speed that you are comfortable with, and allowing up to 30 seconds recovery between drills. As balance and co-ordination develop you will achieve faster feet. To increase the intensity of the exercise, hand-held weights can be used.

Sports vision

Most motorsport drivers look for an edge over their competitors and will quite rightly concentrate on developing their physical and mental fitness to gain that advantage. While there is plenty of material on these aspects of fitness, there remains little in the literature with regard to visual skill, even though it constitutes an integral part of the sport.

Sports vision for a motorsport competitor encompasses a whole host of skills. This includes the obvious visual acuity (acuteness and clearness of sight) as well as accommodation, visual memory, visual search, central-peripheral awareness, vergence, and spatial awareness.

If, as a competitor, you feel that your

concentration fades as the race progresses, or your performance varies considerably especially during night and day, or you have difficulty concentrating on moving objects for sustained periods, or you have visual disturbances, then it is possible that you need to evaluate your sports vision. Try to do this outside the race season, and remember that while some aspects of your deficiencies may be irreversible (for example, colour blindness), almost everything else can be improved upon. The tests and exercises for Sports Vision Training (SVT) are specialised and outside the scope of this book, and competitors should seek expert help from sports optometrists. However, a brief overview of the components of SVT is provided in the panel below.

Andy Blow on top drivers' reaction and response times...

As an athlete myself I have used the Batak machine extensively to improve reactions and peripheral vision. Despite the hours spent practising, my top scores don't compare too well with those of the top F1 and world rally drivers who I've assessed on the machine. Those guys operate at speeds that are quite frankly astonishing!

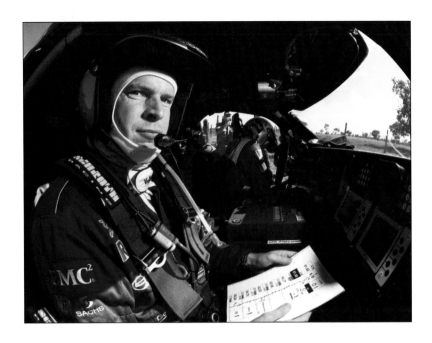

References

Smith, J. F., Bishop, P. A., Ellis, L., Conerly, M. D., Mansfield, E. R. 'Exercise intensity increased by addition of handheld weights to rebounding exercise', *J. Cardiopulm. Rehabil.* 15:34-8.

ABOVE: Rally co-driving requires excellent accommodation skills with constant near to far focusing at high speeds. *(Volkswagen Motorsport/ Red Bull Photofiles)*

Accommodation
Also known as Focus Flexibility, this refers to the ability of the eye to focus on objects from near to far and vice versa. It is an important skill for rally co-drivers who constantly need to cross reference their pace notes (read from less than 1m from their eyes) to the fast moving terrain.

Visual search
This refers to the ability of athletes to extract the relevant information from a situation within a split second. Elite racquet players are able to accurately predict the trajectory of a ball or shuttlecock with simply a glance using this technique while recreational players would spend a long time processing unnecessary information. SVT aims to decrease the time taken for the brain to process information and relay it to the body.

Visual memory
This aspect of sports vision is especially important for motorsport drivers. It relates to the ability of the driver to recall visual information at a glance. Its importance is appreciated during circuit racing where the ability to remember each bend and contour can lead to quicker times and safer driving. This component is a key skill in sports such as cricket where the batting team plays winning shots having recalled the fielding formation of the opposing

team. The Wayne Saccadic Fixator, produced by Wayne Engineering in Illinois, USA, is particularly useful in developing visual memory and is considered by many to be the standard for testing and evaluating a variety of visual skills, including hand-eye coordination, reaction times, and spatial integration.

Spatial awareness
This refers to the body's ability to judge its position or the position of an object relative to itself. Often this is done while the body or the object is moving. This is an important skill, especially in rally driving where the car may need to be set up for a power slide relative to the inside bank without making contact. Spatial awareness is tested with a Brock string, the details of which are beyond the scope of this book.

Central-peripheral awareness
This component of sports vision is especially important in motorsport where the driver has to be acutely aware of his surroundings while focusing on the job of driving. Clearly there is a safety aspect as well.

Vergence
This refers to the ability of the eyes to work together and keep an object in focus irrespective of the distance.

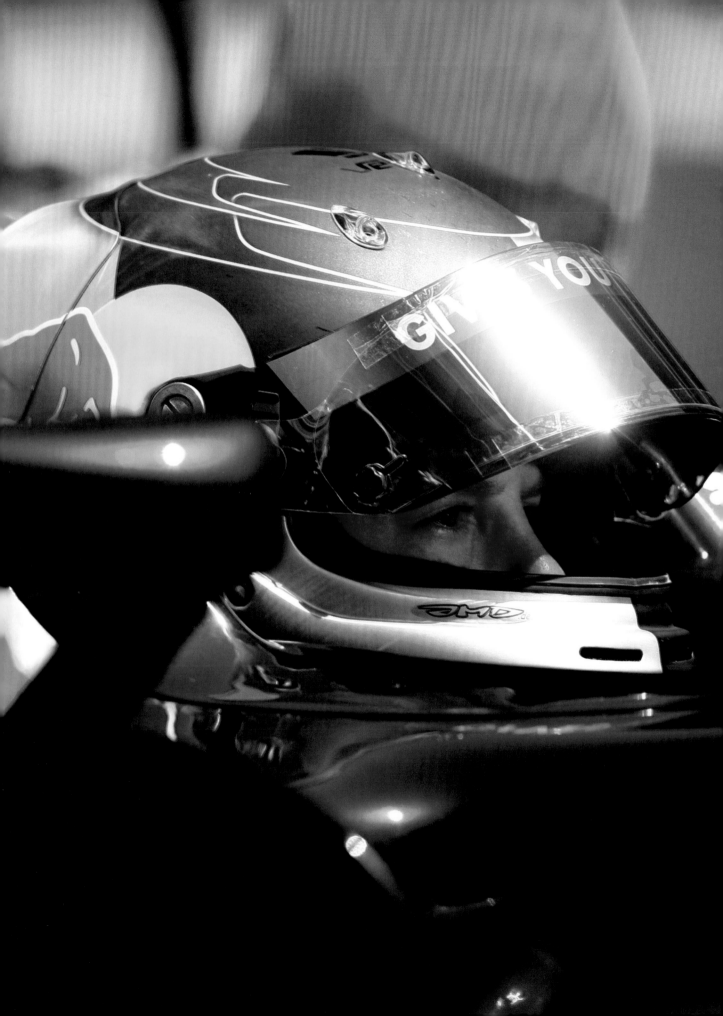

7

Spirit

There is unquestionably a connection between the state of mind and performance of a competitor. This is being more widely recognised, and most top motorsport teams now have sports psychologists who use mental training to help their drivers to achieve peak performance. Most top motorsport drivers now have very similar skills, fitness levels, and competition cars. This means the margin for success is often very slim and not uncommonly down to the competitor who remains focused.

The aim of this chapter is to help you develop a state of mind which makes everything go your way on the day of the event. Some call it being

in the groove, or being in the zone, or on a roll. Whatever it may be called, it is a great feeling of confidence that results in consistent results that may even supersede expectations.

How do you know when you have reached that state of mind? You will be mentally aroused, but just about at the right level. You are relaxed so that your muscles are not tensed up. Your confidence in your own ability and that of your car or kart is such that you expect a reasonable result regardless of what may come your way. You are totally focused on the task in hand and do not allow any distractions to deter you from achieving your goal. You are getting immense enjoyment

OPPOSITE: Sebastian Vettel at the wheel of his Scuderia Torro Rosso. With just minutes to go before the start, this would be a useful time to visualise how the first corner may be taken. *(GEPA Pictures/Red Bull Photofiles)*

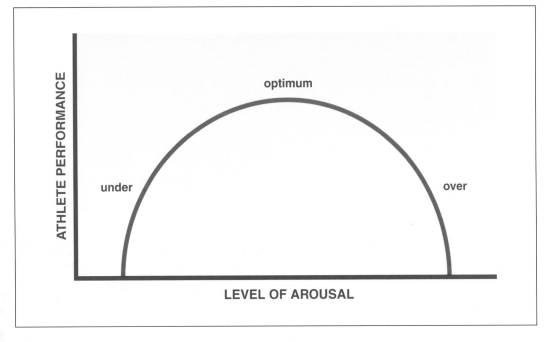

LEFT: The inverted U shape that shows that optimum arousal is achieved by being neither over- nor under-aroused, but in the middle.

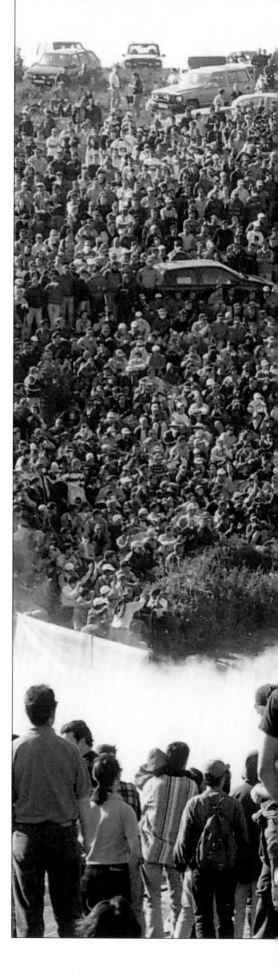

from the race, which seems to be progressing
with minimum *effort* and almost in slow motion
with you fully in *control*. Your racing lines are
smooth and controlled. You hardly notice the
spectators as you are *in charge*!

This is how champion rally-driver Louise Aitken-
Walker felt when she was on a roll:

> *When I was going well, I was going well! I was
> on a song and dance. And nobody could touch
> us. Nobody could beat us. To have that feeling
> was fantastic. It was just exhilarating to drive
> as well as we did. We made history and it was
> great. You believe in yourself and think you can
> do the same again.*

She described how over-arousal can occasionally
lead to problems:

> *Then we had one of our biggest accidents
> ever in Kielder (Forest). Totally wrote off the
> car because we overdid it while on the song
> and dance.*

Your arousal level

For peak performance you need to be at your
optimum level of arousal. Too low or too high a
level will be a hindrance, so it is important that you
know how to hit your personal arousal level. There
are several techniques for doing this and those
commonly used in motorsport are:

- Relaxation
- Imagery including emotional imagery
- Focusing
- Centring
- Positive self-talk
- Target-setting
- Thought stopping.

Relaxation

This is the key to success. You cannot have an
anxious mind in a relaxed body, or the other way
round. However, what is really key is to know
how you interpret feelings of arousal and anxiety,
as you can have different amounts of anxiety in
your mind and in your body. There is even a self-
report tool to help you do this. You need to know
both how much anxiety you have and then how
much that level of anxiety helps or hinders your
performance. If you suffer from a lot of physical
nerves and anxiety, then being able to relax
yourself when you really need to will
radically improve your performance. Up to a
point, physical relaxation techniques can also

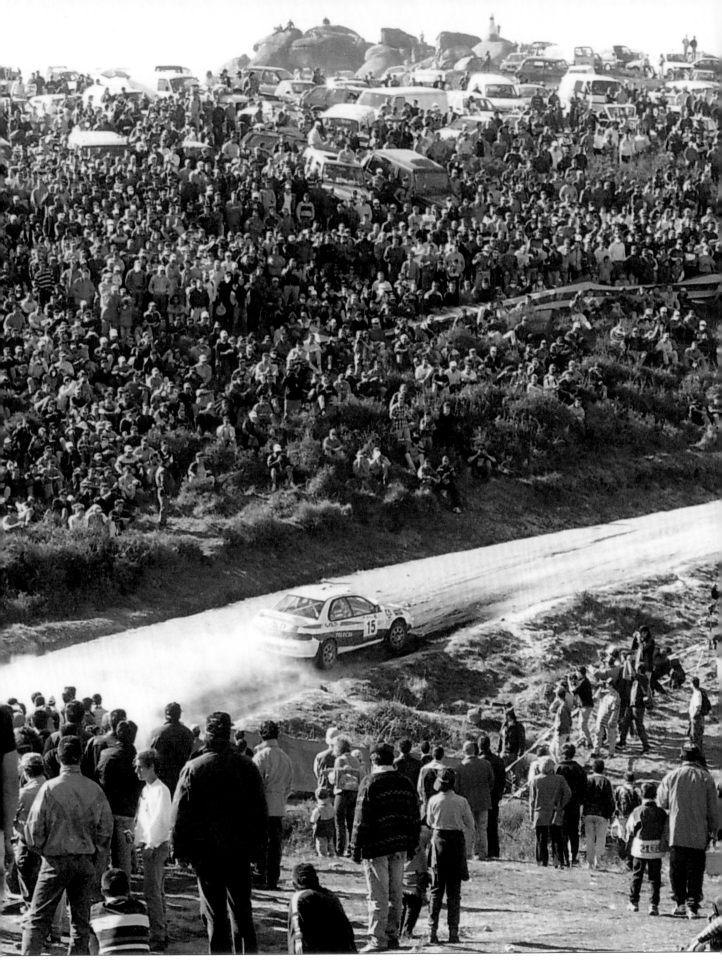

reduce your mental worry, in what is known as a 'crossover effect'.

Several relaxation techniques are available and, as with many things, what is successful for some may not work for others. Try them and stick with one that works for you, but do follow the basic guidelines given below when using your chosen technique. Commonly used techniques include the use of saunas, jacuzzis, hot baths, massage, and music. Massage in particular is useful for physically relaxing tense muscles, and can be used in conjunction with progressive muscle relaxation.

Before you start

- Practice makes perfect. The more you try the technique the more useful it will be.
- Avoid close-fitting clothing and noisy uncomfortable places when practising.
- Lie down if you have to, but avoid falling asleep.
- Enjoy the sessions rather than force yourself to relax.
- Try to empty your mind when relaxing.

Progressive muscle relaxation

There are also many techniques for muscle relaxation. A commonly used one which has proved effective is progressive muscle relaxation. It involves tensing and relaxing muscle groups in sequence. Some start with their toes and move slowly towards their head. Other athletes choose only to relax the muscles they use in competition. For motorsport this is likely to be the upper body with specific attention to the arms, shoulders and neck. By tensing and relaxing each muscle group, competitors will learn to appreciate signals from their bodies. This type of relaxation can be self-taught, or you can follow instructions on one of the commercially available recordings.

Here is a suggested routine:

- Start with five to eight deep breaths while shrugging your shoulders and rolling your head slightly to relax your muscles.
- Then, once you are ready, inhale deeply using your abdominal muscles, and tighten your feet muscles as much as possible and hold for a count of three.
- Relax your muscles as you exhale, and imagine the stress leaving the relaxed muscles.
- Move higher up your body to the calf muscles and repeat the procedure. From there go on to the thighs (front and back), buttocks, abdominal muscles, lower back, chest, upper back,

shoulders, biceps, triceps, forearms, hands, neck, and face muscles.
- As you get better, you can reduce the time to total relaxation and even involve fingers, toes, and other smaller muscles.
- About 20 minutes is a reasonable time to perform total body relaxation for the first time.

A leading F1 Race Engineer (2008) says...

If anything, it's the team staff that need to work on their relaxation, rather than the drivers. As race, data, and vehicle engineers, we have many, many bits of information to process over an extended period and it's tough to keep a clear head. I use both progressive muscle relaxation and centring techniques to moderate arousal and keep me focused and creative. I know my driver benefits from this too. Being able to solve problems is what this job is all about, and I can't do that if my mind is racing.

Imagery

This is an extremely useful technique used by competitors in all sports. Although it is commonly known as visualisation, imagery can in fact use all of the senses. It is best to make use of senses that have the most value to you. This could be any one of imaging a sight, sound, feeling, smell, or some combination. For example, some racers find it easier to imagine sounds rather than sights, and imaging a smell can have a powerful emotional effect, which is helpful when practising this technique. We will continue to use the word 'visualisation', but note that we mean imagery using all of the senses. The technique involves visualising, or seeing, yourself in the race vehicle driving a particular circuit or stage. It is possible that you have already been practising a kind of imagery without being fully aware of it. For instance, when you have an important telephone call to make it is quite likely that beforehand you will practise in your mind what you want to say to give yourself a better chance of ensuring a successful outcome when you actually make the call. It is, effectively, psyching yourself up for the event ahead.

With practice you should be able to develop an emotional state close to what you expect to experience during the race. You will hear the engine revving, feel the force of the acceleration and the change in body position as you drive or power around corners. For some it can be helpful during visualisation to more closely simulate the real thing by adopting the driving position with hands on an imaginary steering wheel and feet on imaginary pedals. This technique is known as functional imagery and is typically more beneficial than simple visualisation.

The Italian Formula 1 driver Giancarlo Fisichella uses imagery as part of his preparation before races. He is able to visualise himself through the entire Monaco circuit with his eyes closed. In doing so he runs through all the gear changes, braking, and acceleration strategies he expects to adopt in the actual race. Amazingly, the timing during these imagery sessions is usually within a few seconds of the practice laps.

Some athletes are known to practise visualisation regularly for ten minutes every week, and as race day draws close they step this up to every day. However, because successful visualisation can arouse emotions as powerful as on the race day itself, it is generally not recommended that you practise it before bedtime! You may find music an excellent motivator and trigger for imagery, but the type of music is important, as loud aggressive music can elicit an inappropriately high arousal level. Imagery is also helpful just before a race to get you into a racing mind.

Emotional imagery

Dealing with emotional setbacks is of massive importance if you're going to progress in motor racing. Distractions and setbacks will hit you week after week, and the drivers who move up the ladder will take both of these in their stride.

In addition to the more understood benefits and methods of imagery mentioned previously, there is a way imagery can be used to improve your emotional reaction to setbacks.

- Find a quiet place where you are away from external distractions.
- Use a form of active relaxation to reduce your mental and physiological arousal to low levels, this should only take up to five minutes, with practice.
- Image the sights, sounds, smells, sensations, and feelings of a setback.
- You may wish to use the imagined example of something that really happened in the past, at which time you did not react favourably to. For example, you became emotionally 'down' and 'withdrawn'. In simple terms, you 'spat the dummy'.
- Imagine reacting favourably to that setback.
- Do this for six days in one week.
- This will upgrade the programming of your sub-conscious, giving you a more effective reaction to the natural setbacks of motor sport.

Harry Tincknell (CR Scuderia) says...
When you're 15-years-old and still in karting, it's very hard not to react badly to setbacks. I've now progressed and am in cars, and find I can deal very well with setbacks, but only because I used mental skills such as imagining myself overcoming problems.

Focusing

Sometimes described as being on auto-pilot, or being connected, or with tunnel vision, focusing is central to competition psychology. It means being relaxed and completely absorbed in your performance. From a safety point of view you are aware of everyone and everything around you, but you don't let the presence of anyone or anything interfere with your concentration.

There are many distractions in motorsport, such as worries about other drivers, the set-up of your car, a bad starting position, stalling on the grid, crashing out, your sponsors' expectations, your personal expectations, and uncertain weather conditions. All these threaten to unnerve you, and the competitors who do best are those who can blot out these distractions and focus on the job in hand.

Like relaxation, focusing comes with practice. The better you get at it the easier it will be to recover from distractions such as spins on the track or road. There are several strategies to help you focus in sport. Not all of them work for everyone, so choose one that suits you and stick with it. Here are some tips to help you focus next time you compete or practise.

- Set out a mental game plan before each event or practice session. When your mind begins to wander, use the plan as a mental cue to help regain focus.
- Be realistic about your targets – your subconscious likes to know that your goals are achievable.
- Your focus will be better if you are physically ready for the race, so practice is important!
- Restore your focus by thinking positively after a setback. For example, following a distracting incident such as a wheel change mid-stage in a rally, reassure yourself that you can complete the rest of the stage in your allotted time, and go for it!
- You obviously enjoy motorsport, and focusing comes much easier when you are enjoying what you are doing. Your enjoyment and focus will be enhanced when you are mentally and physically in peak condition.
- If your focus is starting to drift, remember your

previous best performance. This will remind you of your feeling of success and will stimulate your mind to regain its focus and strive for that feeling again.

- Use visual cues in the car. I know a driver who has a small card with You're The Best! written on it and taped to the sun visor of his race car. Although he knows he is not the best, he uses it as a cue to help him focus while racing. He has, in fact, finished most races he has entered. Such concentration cues could also be verbal, or involve an action, for example clapping your hands or clenching your fist, and so on.

A leading F1 Test Engineer (2008) says…

The young drivers we get coming through to us in F1 very often haven't got all the necessary skills in place. Getting them to concentrate on the right thing at the right time is hugely important. It's too easy for the driver to get distracted away from what matters and then pull the team away with them.

Centring

This is a useful technique to either achieve or regain an optimum arousal level during a race or rally. It takes a few seconds once mastered and relies totally on breathing technique. It is easy to do and is extremely effective after a spin or a crash, for example, where controlling anxiety is crucial. It needs practice, however, to master the technique.

- Make sure you are in quiet and comfortable surroundings and sitting when practising.
- Shrug your shoulders and roll your neck to relax your muscles.
- Start taking a long and deep breath in through your nose using only your abdominal muscles to draw the air in. Try not to use your chest muscles. If your technique is correct, your chest wall will not move as you breathe in.
- Focus at all times on your breathing and on using your abdominal muscles.
- Hold the inhaled breath for a count of two and then slowly exhale for a count of four.

BELOW: The late Richard Burns, 2001 World Rally Champion, can be seen mentally pumping himself at the start of a stage. Imagery, positive self-talk, focusing, and target-setting are all established routines in constant use by all top drivers. *(Mike Gibbon, MVG Photographic)*

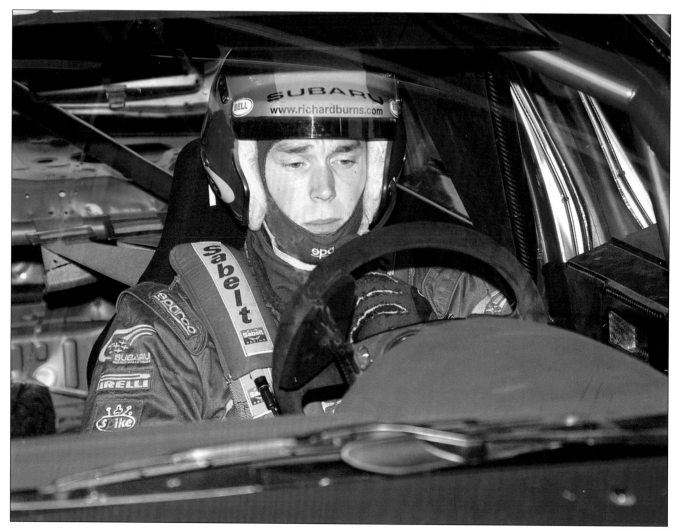

- Do not use any muscles when breathing out – just allow your muscles to relax.
- As you breathe out you will experience a release of tension.
- Repeat the process five to eight times.

Centring should be practised until refocusing is possible with only a single breath and under race conditions. Do make sure, however, when you inhale and exhale that your mind is clear of all distractions.

Positive self-talk

This is a useful tool for regaining the appropriate arousal level. Its purpose is to flush from your mind all negative thoughts, such as 'I will never finish the stage on time' or 'I will never overtake the car ahead!' By using positive self-talk – literally giving yourself a pep talk – you can overcome defeatist feelings and set yourself up to fight back after setbacks.

Target-setting

The value of target-setting is not confined to sport; it's an essential exercise if anything really worthwhile is to be achieved in life. Positive self-talk can also be brought into play by articulating your preset targets during training or practising – for instance: 'I will complete the race circuit in less than three minutes by the end of the afternoon!' Target-setting based on pre-event recce can prove particularly useful in stage rallying. Achieving your stage target times will stimulate your arousal level and will set you up for the following stages.

Thought stopping

In a crossover with other techniques such as positive self-talk, thought stopping, when practised regularly, will give you a handy method for maintaining a positive outlook and a clear and calm head. With such a positive approach, you will be able to trust your vehicle handling skills and not 'get in your own way' with ineffective thinking and resultant behaviour.

This technique is a three-step process:

- First, IDENTIFY your own negative thinking. In time, and with enough quality practice, you will only need to do this step to keep your thoughts on track, as merely being aware of your own thinking will be enough to keep you positive. Note that you cannot hold a positive thought and a negative thought at the same time, it can only be one or the other.

- Second, STOP the negative thought with an appropriate stop signal that has real meaning to you. This will be a sight, sound, feeling (or some combination of all three) depending on what has value to you. You'll need to experiment with a few relevant stop signals before you find one that works. Examples are a waved chequered flag, a large red road stop sign, the sound of being told to stop by someone you know well, etc.
- Third, and finally, REPLACE the previous negative thought with a positive one.

In time you only need do the first two steps, and then finally just the first, to get the required effect. Increased awareness of how you behave and think is key with any sport psychology technique, and thought stopping is fantastic for helping you increase your awareness.

Harry Soden (Team Manager – Connaught Racing Ltd) says...
I run a whole host of karters across many British and Euro series, and a common link with most of them, especially when they're under-16, is that they are very hard on themselves when they make mistakes. They really struggle to remain positive when it's all turning bad. The ones that progress are those that keep a positive but realistic outlook.

Some of the techniques described in this chapter can also be used during your usual training sessions at the gym. For example, having watched a Formula 1 race on television, our man Jim, the amateur rally driver, had a brief imaging session. He realises that he needs to reduce weight for the following season if his performance is to improve, so he sets himself a target weight loss of 1 stone (6kg) over the next three months (target setting) which he achieves with some positive self-talk over the period.

Andy Blow on top drivers mentally preparing for race...
The top drivers in any form of motorsport know exactly how to get themselves into the best frame of mind for racing. I've worked with guys who need to hype themselves up with some light sparring and skipping pre-race, and those who prefer to lie down in the dark for five minutes to relax. Finding out what works for you is the important bit, and you can only do this by learning from your own experiences and trying new ideas.

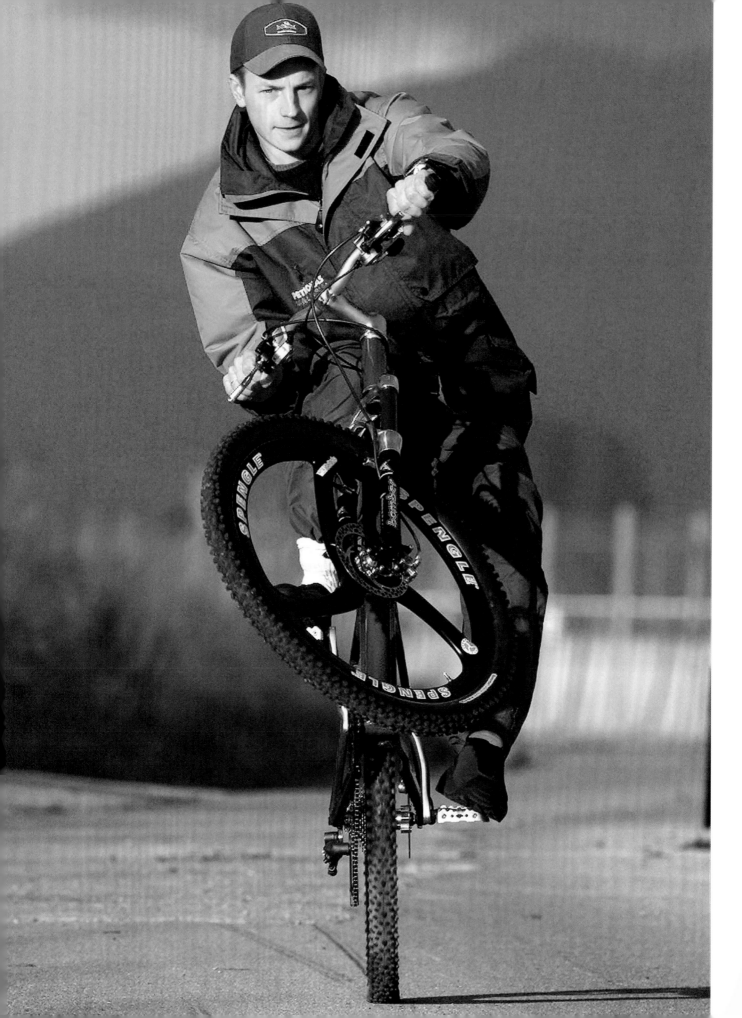

Balance, agility and co-ordination

These three components generally go together in terms of fitness. Evidence suggests they will be invariably developed as you train using the recommendations outlined in the previous chapters. They do, however, deserve special mention as they constitute important qualities that any motorsport competitor must have to be successful. Again, as with strength and skill, these qualities are sport-specific, so by simulating the conditions likely to be encountered in motorsport they can be improved.

Balance

Balance is the ability to keep the body in equilibrium through the co-ordination of all the body sensory systems, including the eyes, ears, and proprioceptive organs such as joints, tendons, and ligaments. There are two types of balance – static and dynamic. Static balance maintains equilibrium in a stationary position, while dynamic balance maintains equilibrium under constantly changing conditions. True enough, some individuals are better at balance than others, but the good news is that it can be improved with training and practice.

The best exercise for balance involves the use of a balance board. Originally devised for skiers and surfers to maintain their skills, the balance board, and latterly the wobble board, are now consistently found in most physiotherapy centres. Their use ranges from post-injury rehabilitation in all age groups to developing sensory integration in disabled people. Before using these boards please obtain professional advice, as falls are dangerous.

Balance can be tested objectively using the Standing Stork Test, undertaken barefooted on the ball of the foot

To perform this test you need the following:
- Flat, non-slip surface.
- Stop-watch.

To undertake the test:
- Place your hands on the hips.
- Stand on one leg.
- Place the non-supported foot against the inside knee of the supporting leg.
- Raise yourself on to the ball of the foot.

To monitor the test:
- Give yourself one minute to practise.
- Start the stop-watch as soon as the heel is raised off the ground.

The test is stopped if:
- The raised heel touches the ground.
- Either hand comes off the hips.
- You hop or swivel the supporting foot to maintain balance.
- The non-supported foot comes off the inside of the knee.

The test is scored as follows:

	Male	Female
Excellent balance	> 50 sec	>30 sec
Good	41-50 sec	23-30 sec
Average	31-40 sec	16-22 sec
Fair	20-30 sec	10-15 sec
Poor	<20 sec	<10 sec

Arnot, R. and Gaines, C., *Sports Talent*, 1984

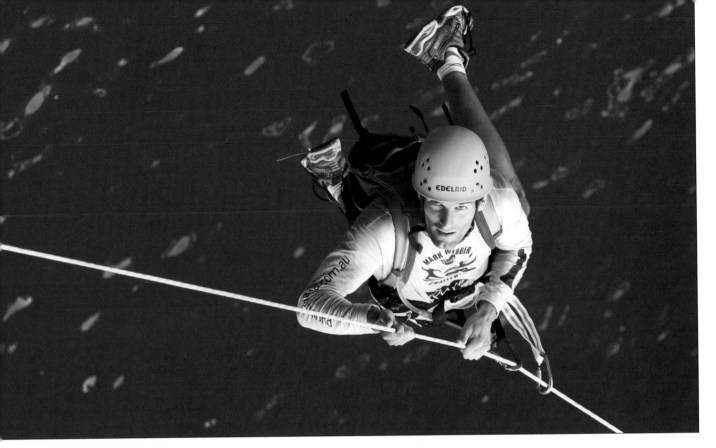

ABOVE: Mark Webber demonstrates why balance, agility and coordination are essential during his annual challenge event. *(www.gettyimages. com)*

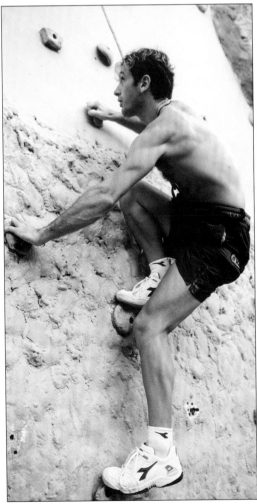

RIGHT: Former Renault driver Jarno Trulli making a strenuous ascent. *(Renault F1)*

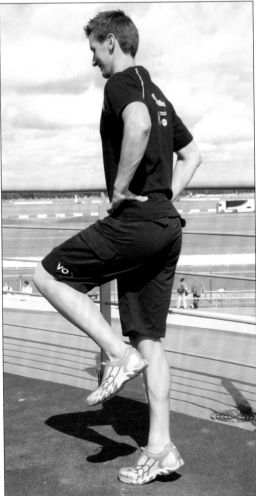

FAR RIGHT: The Standing Stork Test is an objective measure of balance which can be easily performed. *(Dave Blow, myeyefor)*

Agility

Agility is a component that top footballers and racquet players possess and constantly work on to improve. It is how fast the body can change direction and position. Obviously, it must do this gracefully and with balance and co-ordination, or the quality becomes useless.

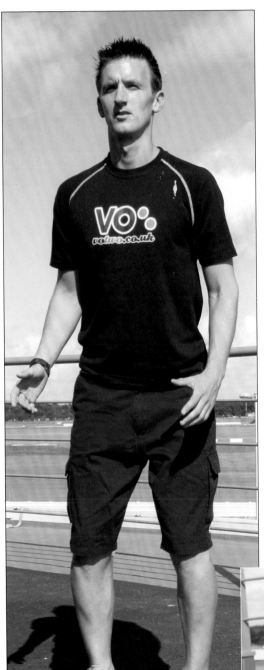

There are several methods of measuring agility, such as the Illinois Agility Run Test, Hexagonal Obstacle Test, and T-Drill Test. The Lateral Change of Direction Test is a simple and reproducible test.

To perform this test you need:
- A flat surface.
- Three cone markers.
- An assistant with a stop-watch

To undertake the test:
- Set the cones in a straight line 5 metres apart.
- Stand by the middle cone.
- The assistant signals the start and which cone to move to (left or right).
- On the signal, move to and touch the indicated cone, go past the middle one to the far cone to touch it and return to the middle.

To measure the test:
- Start the stop-watch on signalling the start.
- Stop the watch when the athlete returns to the middle cone.
- Use the best score in each direction.

The test is scored as follows (based on world-class athletes):

Rank	Females secs	Males secs
91-100	3.22-3.37	2.90-3.05
81-90	3.38-3.53	3.06-3.21
71-80	3.54-3.69	3.22-3.37
61-70	3.70-3.85	3.38-3.53
51-60	3.86-4.01	3.54-3.69
41-50	4.02-4.17	3.70-3.85
31-40	4.18-4.33	3.86-4.01
21-30	4.34-4.49	4.02-4.17
11-20	4.50-4.65	4.18-4.33
01-10	4.66-4.81	4.34-4.49

Chu, D.A., 'Explosive Power and Strength', *Human Kinetics* 1996

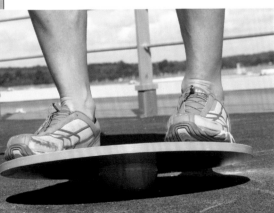

LEFT AND IINSET: The wobble board is encountered in most physiotherapy centres. It is an excellent tool for balance exercises, as well as rehabilitation. *(Dave Blow, myeyefor)*

The agility speed ladder is a good and inexpensive method of developing agility. The following drill is of beginner/medium level and quite simple to perform. Make sure you are adequately warmed up.

- Straddle one side of the ladder with your left foot in first square and your right outside.
- Jump to your left so that your right foot lands in the second square, but keep your left foot in the first square.
- Jump to your right so that your left foot lands in the next square, keeping your right foot in the previous square.
- Repeat the sequence along the ladder.

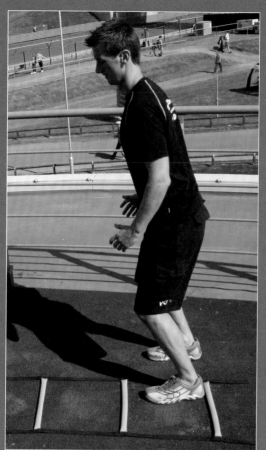
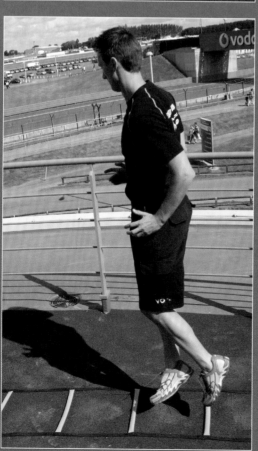
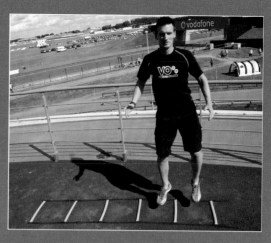
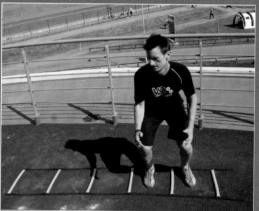
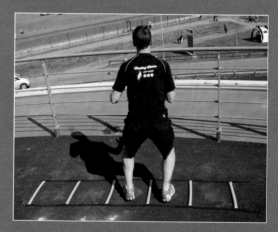
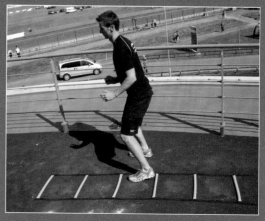

Co-ordination

Co-ordination refers to the smooth execution of the specific task in hand. There is no doubt that this component comes with skill and technique. The more skilful a driver you are, the better coordinated your movements. You apply the power at the right times in the corner; you correct under-steer or over-steer in fluid movements instead of jerky ones that fishtail the car all over the road. Like balance, co-ordination comes with hours of practice. You must expose your body to the same task over and over again so next time it is encountered, you react to it on time, harmoniously, and with poise.

Balance and co-ordination are more important than agility in motorsport. They come with practice and skill and they are best learnt and developed in the race car. It is not the aim of this book to advise you on how to drive a race car, but you will find that these skills are a by-product of training in general, and if you have been following the recommendations in the earlier chapters you will be working on your balance, agility, and co-ordination.

The late 1995 FIA World Rally Champion Colin McRae knew the importance of balance and co-ordination. He enjoyed motorcycling both on and off road. Trail biking is how he first started, and he used it to improve on his fitness and performance.

Andy Blow on agility and coordination skills ...

I was lucky enough to work with Fernando Alonso when he was first test-driving the Renault F1 car several years ago. On a training camp in Kenya I was surprised on a daily basis by his ability level in a wide range of sports that we played, many of which he had never tried before. His natural agility, co-ordination, and will to win was obvious, and it was no surprise that he went on to become a World Champion.

The Hexagonal Obstacle Test is a simple way of testing co-ordination.

To perform this test you need:
- A 66cm hexagon on the floor marked with each side marked A to F.
- An assistant with a stop-watch.

To undertake this test:
- Make sure at all times you face line A.
- Stand in the middle of the hexagon and on the start signal jump with both feet over line B and back to the middle.
- Repeat this with line C through to F at all times facing line A.
- One circuit is complete when you jump over line A.

To measure this test:
- Measure the time taken to complete three circuits.
- After a rest, repeat the test for another three circuits, and average the time for the two tests.

The test must be redone if:
- The wrong line is jumped or you land on a line itself.

The test is scored as follows:

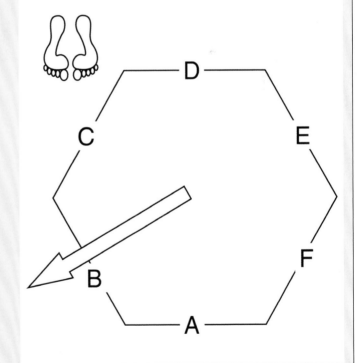

Gender	Excellent	Above average	Average	Below average	Poor
Male	<11.2s	11.2-13.3s	13.4-15.5s	15.6-17.8s	>17.8
Female	<12.2s	12.2-15.3s	15.4-18.5s	18.6-21.8s	>21.8s

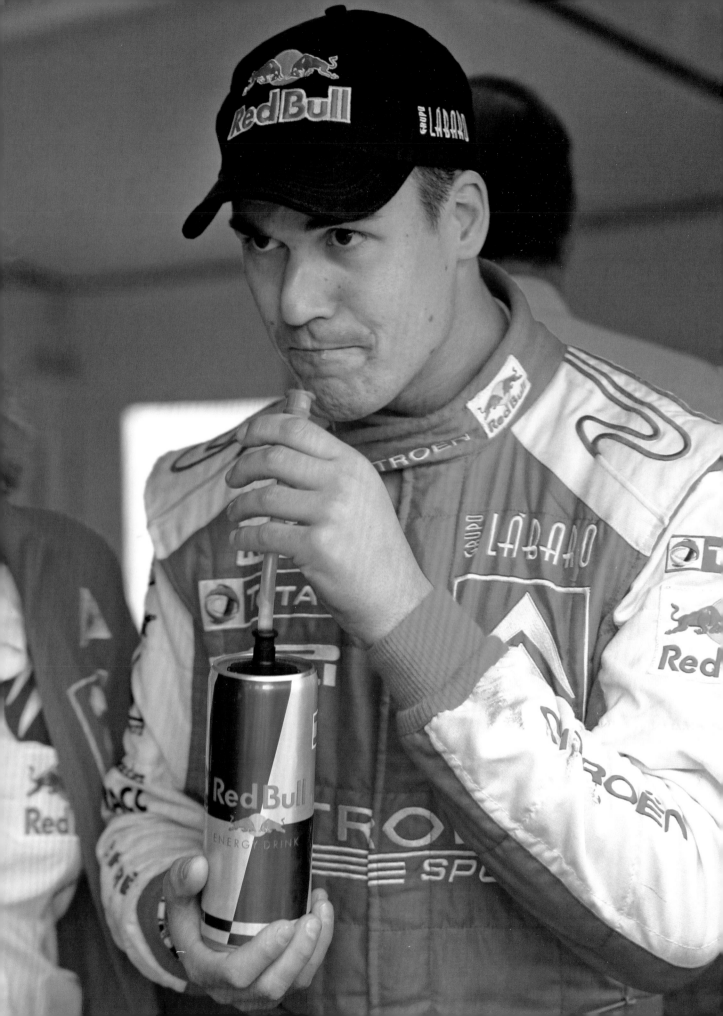

Weight loss and nutrition in motorsport

Lean Machines

There's no doubt that a lighter car will accelerate faster out of corners. However, while competitors often spend vast sums of money shaving extra grams off their equipment in order to gain a competitive edge, they often overlook a less expensive way of giving themselves an advantage – shedding their own body fat! An FIA-approved Kevlar competition seat costs three times as much as a standard fibreglass seat, yet is only 2.5kg (6lb) lighter. This same advantage could be achieved by losing 6lb in body fat a month before a race, and you'd feel leaner and fitter! Dr R. S. Jutley

A few years ago, a basic study evaluating rally drivers at a national event found that as many as half were overweight in relation to their height, some even falling into the medical classification 'obese'. According to the World Health Organisation, obesity is now a serious problem, and the death rate and health problems associated with obesity in the western world now equals that of malnutrition in underdeveloped countries.

So, are you overweight? A quick look at your reflection in a full-length mirror is one indicator – although rather subjective, depending on where you look and how much you pull your tummy in! A more scientific approach is to calculate your Body Mass Index (BMI), which is used by many health professionals to assess health risk.

The ideal BMI is within a range of 19 to 25. A score under 19 suggests you're underweight, while a score over 25 suggests you're overweight. If you have a score over 30, you really need to review your diet and exercise habits, as you would be classified on the BMI scale as obese.

To calculate your BMI, just follow these steps:

- Work out your height in metres.
- Multiply this figure by itself.
- Measure your weight in kilograms (e.g. 75kg).
- Divide your weight by your height squared.

For example, if you're 1.75m and weigh 75kg, you'd calculate your BMI as follows: $75 \div (1.75 \times 1.75) = 24.5$ – just inside the healthy range!

So I'm overweight – how do I lose it?

There is no simple solution, and what works for one person may be a complete disaster for another. Success rates often run low and when people get discouraged they fall back into their bad habits. The

OPPOSITE: Daniel Sordo, upcoming talented WRC driver balances his intake with hydration during stages. *(© Citroën/ McKlein/Red Bull Photofiles)*

BMI	Class
<20	Underweight
20–25	Normal weight
25–30	Overweight
30–40	Obese
>40	Morbidly obese

LEFT: Weight classification according to Body Mass Index.

	5'0"	1"	2"	3"	4"	5"	6"	7"	8"	9"	10"	11"	6'0"	1"	2"	3"	4"	5"	6"	7"	
	49	48	46	45	44	43	42	41	40	39	38	37	36	36	35	34	33	33	32	32 31 30 30 29 29 28 27	110kg
	48	47	46	45	44	43	42	41	40	39	38	37	36	35	34	33	33	32	32	31 30 30 29 28 28 27	109kg
17st –	48	47	46	44	43	42	41	40	39	38	37	36	35	34	33	33	32	31	31	30 29 29 28 28 27	108kg
	48	46	45	44	43	42	41	40	39	38	37	36	35	34	33	33	32	31	30	30 29 28 28 27 27	107kg
	47	46	45	44	42	41	40	39	38	38	37	36	35	34	33	33	33	32 31	31	30 29 29 28 28 27 26	106kg
7lb –	47	45	44	43	42	41	40	39	38	37	36	35	35	34	33	32	32	31	30	30 29 28 28 27 27 26	105kg
	46	45	44	43	42	41	40	39	38	37	36	35	34	34	33	32	31	31	30	29 29 28 28 27 27 26	104kg
	46	45	44	42	41	40	39	38	37	36	36	35	34	33	33	32	31	30	30	29 28 28 27 27 26 26	103kg
16st –	45	44	43	42	41	40	39	38	37	36	35	34	34	33	32	31	30	30	29	28 28 27 27 26 26 25	102kg
	45	44	43	42	40	39	38	38	37	36	35	34	33	33	32	31	30	30	29	29 28 27 27 26 26 25	101kg
	44	43	42	41	40	39	38	37	36	35	35	34	33	32	32	31	30	29	28	28 27 27 26 26 25	100kg
7lb –	44	43	42	41	40	39	38	37	36	35	34	33	33	32	31	30	29	29	28	27 27 26 26 25 25	99kg
	44	42	41	40	39	38	37	36	36	35	34	33	32	31	30	29	28	28	27	27 26 26 25 25 24	98kg
	43	42	41	40	39	38	37	36	35	34	33	33	32	31	30	29	28	28	27	27 26 26 25 25 24	97kg
	43	42	40	39	38	37	37	36	35	34	33	32	32	31	30	29	28	28	27	27 26 26 25 24 24	96kg
15st –	42	41	40	39	38	37	36	35	34	34	33	32	31	31	30	29	28	27	27	26 26 25 25 24 24	95kg
	42	41	40	39	38	37	36	35	34	33	33	32	31	30	30	29	28	27	27	26 25 25 24 24 23	94kg
	41	40	39	38	37	36	35	35	34	33	32	31	31	30	29	29	28	27	27	26 26 25 25 24 23	93kg
7lb –	41	40	39	38	37	36	35	34	33	33	32	31	30	30	29	28	28	27	27	26 25 25 24 23 23	92kg
	40	39	38	37	36	36	35	34	33	32	32	31	30	29	29	28	27	27	26	26 25 25 24 23 22	91kg
	40	39	38	37	36	35	34	34	33	32	31	30	30	29	28	27	27	26	26	25 25 24 24 23 23 22	90kg
14st –	40	39	38	37	36	35	34	33	32	32	31	30	29	29	28	27	27	26	26	25 25 24 24 23 23 22	89kg
	39	38	37	36	35	34	34	33	32	31	30	30	29	28	28	27	26	26	25	25 24 24 23 23 22 22	88kg
	39	38	37	36	35	34	33	32	32	31	30	29	29	28	27	27	26	25	25	24 24 23 23 22 22	87kg
7lb –	38	37	36	35	34	34	33	32	31	30	30	29	28	28	27	27	26	25	25	24 24 23 23 22 22 21	86kg
	38	37	36	35	34	33	32	32	31	30	29	29	28	27	27	26	26	25	25	24 24 23 23 22 22 21	85kg
	37	36	35	34	33	33	32	31	30	30	29	28	28	27	27	26	25	25	24	24 23 23 22 22 21 21	84kg
13st –	37	36	35	34	33	32	32	31	30	29	28	28	27	27	26	26	25	25	24	24 23 23 22 22 21 21	83kg
	36	35	35	34	33	32	31	30	30	29	28	28	27	26	26	25	25	24	24	23 23 22 22 21 21 20	82kg
	36	35	34	33	32	32	31	30	29	29	28	27	27	26	26	25	24	24	23	23 22 22 21 21 20	81kg
	36	35	34	33	32	31	30	30	29	28	28	27	26	26	25	25	24	23	23	22 22 21 21 20 20	80kg
7lb –	35	34	33	32	32	31	30	29	29	28	27	27	26	26	25	24	24	23	23	22 22 21 21 21 20 20	79kg
	35	34	33	32	31	30	30	29	28	28	27	26	26	25	25	24	23	23	22	22 21 21 20 20 19	78kg
	34	33	32	32	31	30	29	29	28	27	27	26	25	25	24	24	23	23	22	22 21 21 20 20 19	77kg
12st –	34	33	32	31	30	30	29	28	28	27	26	26	25	25	24	23	23	22	22	21 21 20 20 19 19	76kg
	33	32	32	31	30	29	28	28	27	27	26	25	25	24	24	23	23	22	22	21 21 20 20 19 19	75kg
	33	32	31	30	30	29	28	28	27	26	26	25	24	24	23	23	22	22	21	21 20 20 20 19 19 18	74kg
7lb –	32	32	31	30	29	29	28	27	26	26	25	24	24	23	23	22	22	21	21	20 20 19 19 19 18	73kg
	32	31	30	30	29	28	27	27	26	26	25	24	24	23	23	22	22	21	21	20 20 19 19 18 18	72kg
	32	31	30	29	28	28	27	26	26	25	24	24	23	23	22	22	21	21	20	20 19 19 18 18 18	71kg
11st –	31	30	30	29	28	27	27	26	25	25	24	24	23	23	22	22	21	20	20	19 19 19 18 18 17	70kg
	31	30	29	28	28	27	26	26	25	24	24	23	23	22	22	21	21	20	20	19 19 18 18 18 17	69kg
	30	29	29	28	27	27	26	25	25	24	24	23	22	22	21	21	20	20	19	18 18 18 17 17	68kg
7lb –	30	29	28	28	27	26	26	25	24	24	23	23	22	22	21	20	20	19	19	19 18 18 17 17 17	67kg
	29	29	28	27	26	26	25	24	24	23	23	22	22	21	21	20	20	19	19	18 18 17 17 16	66kg
	29	28	27	27	26	25	25	24	24	23	22	22	21	21	20	20	19	19	18	18 18 17 17 16 16	65kg
10st –	28	28	27	26	26	25	24	24	23	23	22	22	21	20	20	19	19	18	18	18 17 17 16 16	64kg
	28	27	27	26	25	24	24	23	23	22	22	21	20	20	19	19	18	18	17	17 17 16 16 16	63kg
	28	27	26	25	25	24	24	23	22	22	21	21	20	20	19	19	18	18	17	17 16 16 16 15	62kg
7lb –	27	26	26	25	24	24	23	23	22	22	21	20	20	19	19	18	18	17	17	17 16 16 16 15	61kg
	27	26	25	24	24	23	23	22	22	21	21	20	20	19	19	18	18	17	17	16 16 16 15 15	60kg
	26	26	25	24	24	23	22	22	21	21	20	20	19	19	18	18	17	17	16	16 16 15 15 15	59kg
9st –	26	25	24	24	23	23	22	22	21	20	20	19	19	18	18	17	17	16	16	16 15 15 15 14	58kg
	25	25	24	23	23	22	22	21	21	20	20	19	18	18	18	17	17	16	16	15 15 15 15 14	57kg
	25	24	24	23	22	22	21	21	20	20	19	19	18	18	17	17	16	16	16	15 15 15 14 14	56kg
7lb –	24	24	23	23	22	21	21	20	20	19	19	19	18	18	17	17	16	16	15	15 15 14 14 14	55kg
	24	23	23	22	22	21	21	20	20	19	19	18	18	17	17	16	16	15	15	14 14 14 13	54kg
	24	23	22	22	21	21	20	20	19	19	18	18	17	17	16	16	16	15	15	14 14 14 14 13	53kg
8st –	23	23	22	21	21	20	20	19	19	18	18	18	17	17	16	16	16	15	15	14 14 14 13 13	52kg

ABOVE: A Body Mass Index chart extracted from the 'Body Mass Index Ready Reckoner' published by Servier Laboratories Ltd. Find your height in metres or feet and inches and your weight in kilograms or stones. The two readings meet at your BMI. *(Courtesy: Servier Laboratories Limited 1997)*

Legend:
- very obese
- obese
- overweight
- healthy
- underweight

Is my excess weight fat?

- Most people believe that extra weight is extra fat. This is not the case at all. Body weight consists of lean tissue and body fat. Lean tissue is made up of water, muscle, organs, and blood; and fat simply consists of FAT! The proportion of fat is affected by an individual's level of fitness.

- The inactive and overweight competitor who eats a high-fat diet is likely to have an extra weight value that is mainly made up of fat rather than lean tissue. On the other hand, an active competitor on a relatively balanced diet who is overweight is likely to have more lean tissue than fat to account for the extra weight. If you really want to know how much fat you are carrying, then body composition measurements are necessary.

- Many health and fitness clubs will measure body composition using skin fold callipers or bio-electrical impedance analysis (BIA). The callipers measure fat just underneath the skin at various places on the body, such as the hip area, the biceps, triceps and shoulder blade, among others. Using these measurements and other calculations, body fat percentages can be calculated.

- BIA uses a small electric current that passes through the body. The fat cells act as a resistance to the current, while lean tissue is a good conductor of the current. The amount of resistance gives an indication of percentage of body fat. Make sure you are well hydrated when having a BIA measurement, otherwise you will read a higher percentage body fat. There is no ideal body fat percentage. Different sports require different percentages, but in motorsport it is probably important that you stay as low as possible without compromising on other components of fitness. As a general guide, the percentage associated with the lowest health risk is 13-18% in males and 18-25% in females.

- There are more accurate means for calculating body fat but these are rarely found outside research centres and hospitals.

consolation is that the principles for losing weight are really simple and can be applied easily. There are literally hundreds of health and fitness plans available from self-professed experts on weight loss, many of which are based on poor scientific principles. And the introduction of the Internet into everyday life has done little more than to increase the confusion that already exists.

Put very simply, for weight loss to occur, energy expenditure (energy used by the body) must be greater than energy intake (food and drink consumed). This must be for a reasonably prolonged period of time and must result in the creation of an energy deficit.

One sure way of creating an energy deficit is to reduce or modify input. To better understand this, it is important to have a working knowledge of Resting Metabolic Rate (RMR). This is the number of calories the body must have per day to keep essential body functions ticking over. RMR varies according to age and sex. To estimate your RMR use the table in *Fig. 1*.

RMR calculates the number of calories required assuming you are lying in bed for 24 hours doing nothing. Most people do not do that, so the actual number of calories required per day varies according to their lifestyle. Those who are very active (labourers) generally need twice the RMR. To estimate your daily energy expenditure use the table in *Fig 2*.

Jim weighs 85kg and wants to lose weight for the following season. He is a garage owner who runs the business largely from behind a desk. He does, however, make regular visits to the working area during the day. From the table in *Fig. 1* his RMR is (85 x 11.6) + 879 = 1,865 calories (kcal). Given his lifestyle, his daily expenditure is 1,865 x 1.7 = 3,170kcal. To lose weight he must consume food and fluid that has a total calorie count of less than 3,170kcal in 24 hours.

Drastically reducing the calorie intake is not good for the body and does not shed fat any faster. The body will recognise such a drop in calorie intake as a sign of starvation and will begin to break down lean tissue instead of fat. The ideal method is to cut the daily calorie count by 15% and no more.

So, Jim needs to consume 85% x 3,170 = 2,695kcal every day for fat loss to occur. Reducing calorie intake is only part of the game. The diet must also be modified to give a healthy balance of carbohydrate, fat, protein, and other essential components. What's given here is a general guide only. The general rule of thumb in motorsport is that the leaner and lighter the competitor, the faster he or she will be. However,

RESTING METABOLIC RATE CALCULATOR

Age (years)	Male	Female
10–17	(wt in kg x 17.5) + 651	(wt in kg x 12.2) + 746
18–29	(wt in kg x 15.3) + 679	(wt in kg x 14.7) + 496
30–59	(wt in kg x 11.6) + 879	(wt in kg x 8.7) + 829

ABOVE: Fig. 1. Use this table to calculate what your daily Resting Metabolic Rate (RMR) should be in kcal. *(Taken from 1985 FAO/ WHO/UNO report)*

it is very important that weight loss occurs in a controlled way and doesn't happen too quickly (no more than 1/2 lb (225g) per day).

More information on the subject can be obtained from books on nutrition or from recognised websites such as the Calorie Control Council. This organisation uses sound scientific research as a cornerstone to their published work which may be found on www.caloriecontrol.org.

What makes a healthy diet?

A healthy diet should be made up of a balance of carbohydrates, protein, and healthy fats, as well as a wide range of vitamins and minerals.

Proteins are essential for growth and repair of body tissue, and are provided by meat, fish, eggs, beans, nuts, and seeds. Unless you're doing really strenuous aerobic exercise, you shouldn't need to supplement your protein, as a balanced diet should provide adequate amounts for most people who take part in sport.

Healthy fats, known technically as 'unsaturated fats', are an important source of energy and a major component of cell membranes. Unsaturated fats can be subdivided into 'monounsaturated' fats and 'polyunsaturated' fats. Monounsaturated fats are found in avocados, nuts, and plant oils, such as olive oil. Polyunsaturated fats consist of two main types: omega-3 fatty acids (available in oily fish, such as salmon, tuna, herring, mackerel, and sardines) and omega-6 fatty acids (found in vegetable oils. such as sunflower and corn oil). The fats to avoid are saturated fats, which are found in red meat, dairy products, and cakes.

BELOW: Fig. 2. Daily Energy Expenditure is calculated by multiplying your RMR by a factor depending upon your level of activity during the day.

DAILY ENERGY EXPENDITURE

Level of daily activity	Daily expenditure
Light (e.g. office job)	RMR x 1.55
Moderate (e.g. regular walking during day)	RMR x 1.7
Heavy (e.g. labouring)	RMR x 2.0

There are a great many different vitamins and minerals, but it is essential that we include in our diet as many as possible, since they are necessary components of the myriad of biochemical processes that take place inside us each and every day. The best way to ensure that we get the required vitamins and minerals is to eat a wide variety of fruit and vegetables. We're all familiar with the phrase '5-a-day', but it is important to understand that this is the minimum recommendation. Someone serious about sport should really be aiming for ten different fruit and vegetables a day, and to try to vary each type from one day to the next.

Carbohydrates are converted by the body into glucose and glycogen. During exercise, our muscles are fuelled by glucose in the blood, and glycogen stored in the liver and in the muscles themselves. Glucose and glycogen are inter-convertible. This means that if the body has enough glucose, carbohydrates will be converted into glycogen, while if there is a shortage glycogen will be turned into glucose. Adequate consumption of carbohydrates is vital in order to maintain the balance between glucose in the blood and glycogen in the liver and muscles.

Carbohydrates fuel all activities, and it is important to choose them wisely in order to avoid peaks and troughs of energy. The best ones are complex carbohydrates (such as oats, rice, potatoes, and wheat-free bread or pasta). Being starchy and fibrous, complex carbohydrates release their energy slowly and steadily into the bloodstream. This is in contrast to simple carbohydrates (the sugars found in chocolates, cakes, and fizzy drinks) which release their energy quickly, leading to 'peaks' of energy followed by 'troughs' of lethargy.

A measure of how quickly the energy of carbohydrates is made available for use by the body is its glycaemic index (GI). Generally, high GI foods are digested quickly and release their glucose quickly to produce a fast energy boost. In contrast, foods with a lower GI take longer to break down and tend to increase glycogen reserves rather than meet instant energy needs.

Foods with a low GI

■ Grains
All Bran, barley, buckwheat, bulgur wheat, grain breads, oat bran, oats, pasta, pumpernickel, rice noodles, seeded breads, sourdough rye

■ Vegetables and pulses
Baked beans, black-eyed peas, butter beans, chickpeas, haricot beans, kidney beans, lentils, lima beans, peas, new potatoes, soya beans, sweet potatoes, sweet corn, radishes, lettuce, cucumber

■ Fruit
Apples, bananas, cherries, dried apples, dried apricots, grapefruit, grapes, kiwi fruit, oranges, peaches, pears, plums, prunes, strawberries, raspberries, tomatoes

■ Snack Food
Apple juice, cashew nuts, corn chips, hot chocolate, peanuts, flapjacks, fruit, popcorn

Foods with a medium GI

■ Grains
Arborio rice, arrowroot biscuits, basmati rice, brown rice, chapatti, couscous, croissants, gnocchi, melba toast, pita bread, wholemeal bread

■ Vegetables and pulses
Beetroot, broccoli, carrots, potatoes

■ Fruit
Dried figs, melon, pineapple, apricots, peaches, mango

■ Snack foods
Digestive biscuits, ice cream, muesli bars, muffins, crisps, raisins, cake, cookies

Foods with a high GI

■ Grains
Baguettes, bagels, bread stuffing, coco pops, corn pops, crackers, crunchy nut cornflakes, white rice, tapioca, Rice Krispies, white pasta

■ Vegetables, Pulses, and Fruit
Broad beans, jacket potatoes, mashed potato, pumpkin, swede, parsnips, dates, watermelon

■ Snack Foods
Doughnuts, French fries, fruit bars, honey, glucose tablets, jelly beans, scones, waffles

Keeping a Food Diary

If you are serious about eating healthily, then record a food diary for a few days. Write down everything you eat and drink, and the times of consumption as well.

Let's take a look at Jim's diary for the day:

There are several problems with Jim's diet
- ■ Too many calories considering his lifestyle.
- ■ Too much fat. He is eating a lot of 'hidden fat' in the burgers, bacon roll, and fries.
- ■ Too little fibre. 30g per day is recommended, especially if trying to lose weight. High-fibre foods tend to be low in fat and also give the 'full belly' feeling.
- ■ Too little fluid. Coffee and alcohol dehydrate the body. Colas tend to have little or no nutrients.
- ■ Poor timing of meals. A high RMR is best maintained by eating regularly during the day instead of eating heavily at night as Jim does.

MONDAY	(TUESDAY)	WEDNESDAY	THURSDAY	FRIDAY	SATURDAY	SUNDAY

Breakfast

Time: ....

....

....

....

....

Lunch

Time: ....

....

....

....

....

Dinner

Time: ....

....

....

....

....

Snacks/Treats

.... Time: ....

.... Time: ....

.... Time: ....

.... Time: ....

Drinks

....

....

....

....

MONDAY	TUESDAY	(WEDNESDAY)	THURSDAY	FRIDAY	SATURDAY	SUNDAY

Breakfast

Time: 07.30

Bacon roll

....

....

....

Lunch

Time: 13.00

Fast-food burger

French fries

Apple pie

....

Dinner

Time: 20.30

Chicken curry

Naan bread

Onion Pakoras

....

Snacks/Treats

Cookies (2) .... Time: 11.00

Iced bun .... Time: 16.00

.... Time: ....

.... Time: ....

Drinks

Coffee with 2 sugars (breakfast)

Fizzy Cola drink (mid-morning snack)

Coffee with 2 sugars (mid-afternoon)

Bottled beer (1) with dinner

Hydration

Occupying around 70% of your body mass, water is the most plentiful substance in your body. It is required by each of your body's millions of cells and is essential in transporting nutrients, removing waste and regulating body temperature. With such an important role, it is surprising how few people drink enough water throughout the day. It is interesting to note that a deficiency of just 1% of water can cause headaches and other aches and pains, yet people rarely realise that the solution is so simple – drinking enough water! We should aim to drink 2 litres a day as a minimum, and about 250ml every 30 minutes when exercising. See 'Isotonic drinks' in Chapter 11 for an important kind of sports drink.

One very common obstacle in the way of drinking the required amount of water is to mistake thirst for hunger. Another is to choose a coffee, tea or fizzy drink when what you actually need is a glass of pure water. Nowadays people don't think twice about topping up with fluids containing a concoction of things such as sugar, sweeteners, caffeine, gas, preservatives, and salt. Motor sport enthusiasts wouldn't dream of putting the automotive equivalent of fizzy drinks in their cars or motorbikes, yet they do it to their bodies a lot of the time!

Secrets of hydration

- The rate of passage of water from your stomach to your intestines depends on how much water is actually in your stomach. If there is lots of fluid, then it is like a flood flowing from your stomach to the intestines. The idea is to have a smaller amount of water so it drips like a tap into the intestines. So practise sipping often throughout the day. Take 3-4 sips of water every ten minutes or so.

- If you're going to be exercising for less than 60 minutes, don't worry about putting carbohydrates in your drinks – plain water is fine. However, for prolonged exercise it is advisable to add a carbohydrate.

- Cold drinks are absorbed no more quickly than warm drinks. However, cold drinks are often more palatable than warm ones during exercise. So, if cold drinks help you to drink large quantities of fluid while you exercise, stick with cold drinks!

Good Hydrators: water, isotonic drinks, juices, herbal teas
Bad Hydrators: tea, coffee, fizzy drinks, alcohol

There is more information on hydration, and how to make your own drinks in Chapter 11.

Supplementation

Although everyone eating a good diet should – in theory – get sufficient nutrients from their food, there are three reasons why Barbara Cox, leading nutritionist and CEO of Nutrichef, advises people to take a good multi-vitamin and mineral supplement:

- Nowadays, soil is being depleted of minerals and vitamins due to over-farming.
- Fruit and vegetables are often picked before the ripening stage when minerals and vitamins are formed.
- The minerals and vitamins that were present when the fruit and vegetables were picked may well have broken down by the time the produce reaches the supermarket shelves.

On the basis of the above, Barbara Cox recommends the following for motorsport competitors:

- A good quality multi-vitamin and mineral supplement.
- Antioxidant supplementation.
- Omega-3 supplementation.

Taking a high quality multi-vitamin is like having an insurance policy against possible vitamin and mineral deficiencies. Antioxidants ward off free-radical damage that can be caused by a poor diet and stress, and they can also counteract the increase in free radicals produced as a result of exercise (Packer, L., *Med. Sci. Sports* 1989 21:42-47). As for an omega supplement, research shows that flaxseed oil can prevent and alleviate post-exercise fatigue and accelerate recovery. It has also been reported that it may improve athletic performance (Luoma, 'EFAs', *Muscle Media*, 1997, 64:62-68).

100 Star Foods

Barbara Cox, leading food nutritionist and co-author of this chapter says:

I was fortunate enough to live in Japan for eight years, where I became interested in healthy eating. I was particularly struck by the huge variety of different kinds of food eaten in a typical week, and I believe that the consequent variety of nutrients is one of the reasons why Japan has lower levels of cancer and heart disease than in the west. Looking into this further, I found that the Japanese eat an average of 100 different kinds of food a week, which is in stark contrast to the UK average of just 20.

The advantage that the Japanese have with this wide variety of different foods is that they are much more likely to be giving themselves the full complement of nutrients (especially all the different vitamins and minerals) that we need as raw material for all of our different biochemical processes. In contrast, we in the West tend to stay within the same food groups and choices, thus limiting our chances of consuming the full scale of nutrients that we need.

Below is a list of perhaps the best 100 ingredients on the planet. Count how many of them you consumed in the past seven days!

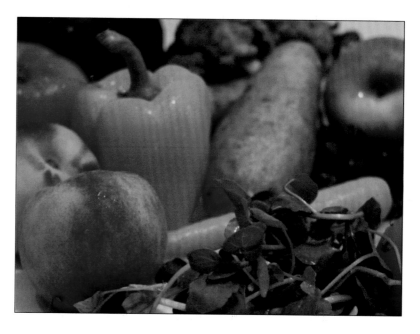

FRUIT AND VEGETABLES

The basics

1. **Red and orange peppers.** Rich in disease-fighting antioxidants; they contain three times as much vitamin C as citrus fruit, and have antibacterial qualities.
2. **Broccoli.** A cancer-fighting vegetable high in calcium, folate, and antioxidants.
3. **Carrots.** They have cholesterol-lowering properties and are rich in vitamin A, which is necessary for healthy eyes.
4. **Sweet potatoes.** Rich in fibre, vitamin A, vitamin C, folate, iron, copper, and calcium.
5. **Watercress.** Packed with folate, iron and beta-carotene, they are good for cardiovascular and thyroid function.
6. **Tomatoes.** Packed with vitamin C and the antioxidant lycopene.
7. **Red cabbage.** Rich in fibre, vitamin C, beta-carotene, and disease-fighting sulphorane. It is detoxifying, too, and helps support the liver.
8. **Blueberries.** Loaded with anthocyans, vitamin C, and fibre. They're expensive but they have the highest rate of antioxidants of any readily available fruit.
9. **Apples.** Rich in vitamin C and soluble fibre, which is gentler on your gut than insoluble fibre.
10. **Peaches.** Easily digested, they have a cleansing effect on your kidneys and bladder, too.

Super boosters

11. **Asparagus.** High in nutrients, especially vitamin K (important for blood clotting), and folic acid. A good liver tonic.

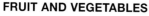

12. **Beansprouts.** Rich in vitamin B3, which keeps down cholesterol levels and regulates blood sugar. Also rich in biochemicals that aid digestion.
13. **Aubergines.** Full of calcium and beta-carotene, they are good for the circulatory system.
14. **Mange-Tout.** Good source of fibre and are rich in vitamins A, C, and K.
15. **Watermelon.** A powerful anti-ager that's rich in lycopene and immunity-boosting vitamin C.
16. **Pineapple.** Contains bromelain, an important digestive enzyme that kills bacteria. It's an anti-bloat food, too.
17. **Raspberries.** A good detox fruit, a serving of which provides 43% of your daily dose of vitamin C, as well as other powerful antioxidants.
18. **Kiwi fruit.** Very rich in immunity-boosting vitamin C, magnesium and potassium, which are vital for healthy nerves and muscles. One kiwi contains your reference nutrient intake of vitamin C.
19. **Cranberries.** Rich in anti-ageing antioxidants that help prevent the build-up of plaque in the arteries, and may help to prevent urinary tract infections.
20. **Pomegranate.** Hailed as a new super fruit, thanks to high levels of vitamins A, C, and E, and other antioxidants. May well help ward off heart disease.
21. **Goji berries.** These Asian fruits contain up to 21 trace minerals. They're said to be, of all known foods, the richest source of carotenoids, including beta-carotene. Available as dried fruits from health food shops.

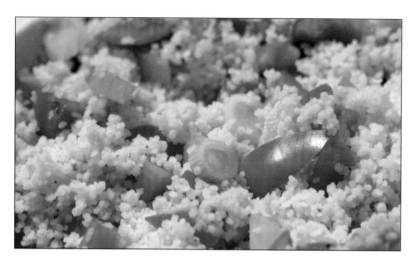

CARBOHYDRATES

22. **Brown rice.** Good source of energy, as well as B vitamins.
23. **Pearl barley.** Linked with lower cholesterol levels, it is good for the digestive tract and contains zinc, which boosts the immune system.
24. **Oats.** A superb source of energy and fibre, oats reduce cholesterol and are packed with minerals and vitamin B5 – important for hair, skin, and nails.
25. **Quinoa.** Good source of protein, vitamin E, iron, and zinc, which is good for the immune system.
26. **Spelt.** A distant relative of wheat, but it's more easily absorbed by the body.
27. **Rye.** Contains iron and B vitamins. Regular intakes of rye are linked with lower rates of heart disease.
28. **Buckwheat.** High in protein; use this gluten-free grain in flour form for bread, pancakes, etc.
29. **Millet.** This gluten-free carbohydrate is great as an alternative to rice. It contains zinc, iron, and vitamins B3 and E.
30. **Soba noodles.** Usually made from buckwheat, they may have wheat flour added. They contain selenium and zinc.
31. **Couscous.** A source of slow release carbohydrate, it's rich in vitamin B3, which provides energy. It's also rich in minerals and vitamin B5, which is important for healthy hair, skin, and nails.
32. **Bulgur/cracked wheat.** Both are good sources of slow-release carbohydrates.

PROTEIN
The basics
33. **Walnuts.** A good source of omega-3 and antioxidants.

34. **Shellfish.** Most varieties are high in omega-3, fatty acids, and zinc.
35. **Turkey.** A rich source of vitamin B12, potassium, zinc, and iron.
36. **Chickpeas.** Rich in phyto-oestrogens, which are linked with lower rates of some cancers.
37. **Eggs.** One egg provides a third of your need for vitamin B12, which is essential for the nervous system.
38. **Kidney beans.** A great source of fibre, and rich in complex carbohydrates.
39. **Tofu.** A low-fat protein that contains some iron, zinc, and B vitamins.
40. **Mackerel.** The richest fish source of omega-3s!
41. **Edamame.** A soya bean that's rich in cancer-fighting isoflavones.
42. **Venison.** Lower in saturated fats than other red meats.

Super boosters
43. **Mussels.** Provide an excellent supply of B12. Rich in selenium and iodine, which helps thyroid function.
44. **Mung beans.** Most nutritious when sprouted, they're rich in minerals, phyto-oestrogens, and vitamin C.
45. **Rabbit.** Lower in fat than other red meats and is rich in iron, zinc, and vitamin B12.
46. **Pumpkin seeds.** A particularly good source of iron and zinc.
47. **Dulse (seaweed).** High in vitamin B, iron, and potassium.

SEASONAL PRODUCE

48. **Artichoke.** Rich in fibre, vitamin C, potassium, and magnesium, they're good for digestion.
49. **Acorn squash.** Packed with nutrients that benefit your eyes, blood pressure, and immunity.
50. **Celeriac.** Contains potassium, phosphorus, vitamin C, and fibre. Celeriac is good for regulating blood pressure.
51. **Beetroot.** High in vitamin C, beta-carotene, magnesium, iron, and folic acid. Beetroot is great for detoxing the liver.
52. **Red onion.** Rich in cancer-fighting quercetin, and a great detoxifier.
53. **Brussels sprouts.** Loaded with folic acid, vitamin C, and vitamin K.
54. **Passion fruit.** A good source of vitamins A and C; thought to aid sleep.
55. **Satsumas.** Excellent source of vitamin C and folate.
56. **Kale.** Full of iron and folic acid, and easy to use in stir-fries.

FATS AND OILS

Healthy fats are important for your metabolism and absorption of vitamins A, D, E, and K. They are also good for brain development and for telling you when you've had enough to eat! Aim for no more than 70g a day.

57. **Flaxseed oil.** Rich in fatty acids thought to prevent heart disease.
58. **Rapeseed oil.** A healthy cooking oil and a source of omega-3s.
59. **Avocado.** Contains vitamin E, so it's great for your skin.
60. **Olive oil.** Rich in oleic acid, which helps you absorb omega-3s.
61. **Hazelnut oil.** High in omega-9s and contains vitamin E.

HERBS AND SPICES

62. **Ginger.** Good for digestion and is also an anti-inflammatory.
63. **Garlic.** This has antibacterial, antiviral, and antiseptic qualities.
64. **Mint.** Contains vitamin C, calcium, and iron.
65. **Turmeric.** Containing curcumin, it has anti-inflammatory and cancer-fighting effects.
66. **Cinnamon.** A warming spice, useful for treating colds, stomach pains, and poor circulation.
67. **Bay leaves.** They provide traces of iron and phosphorus, and are good for digestion.
68. **Rosemary.** A good stimulant for your immune system and a powerful antioxidant.
69. **Chives.** These contain compounds that may help to lower blood cholesterol levels.
70. **Coriander.** A good tonic for your stomach, heart, and urinary tract.
71. **Dill.** Antibacterial herb that's a good source of calcium.
72. **Fennel.** Known for its diuretic effects, it's traditionally used to relieve intestinal cramps.
73. **Parsley.** Contains vitamin C, folic acid, and beta-carotene.
74. **Sage.** This is an anti-inflammatory and is good for digestion.
75. **Thyme.** Known best for its antioxidant properties.

PLUS...
PMS BEATERS

76. **Sunflower and pumpkin seeds.** These help beat inflammation.
77. **Porridge.** Its slow-release energy may help control sugar cravings.
78. **Bananas.** Contain serotonin, which boosts mood, while their potassium may help beat fluid retention, too.

79. **Lentils.** Loaded with magnesium – low levels of which may cause cramps.
80. **Wholegrains.** Rich in vitamin B6 and B1, which help beat cramps.
81. **Celery.** Contains phytochemicals that may help calm nerves.
82. **Spinach.** Rich in folate – low levels of which have been linked to depression.

ANTI-AGERS

83. **Green tea.** Rich in catechin polyphenols, which slow the ageing process.
84. **Pink grapefruit.** Contains lycopene, which mops up free radicals.
85. **Salmon.** Contains dimethylaminoethanol, a substance found to stimulate memory and cognitive function.

BRAIN FEEDERS

86. **Basil.** Used by herbalists for its antidepressant properties.
87. **Strawberries.** Rich in antioxidants that are said to aid concentration.
88. **Yeast extracts.** Filled with brain-boosting B vitamins.
89. **Sardines.** Bursting with omega-3 fatty acids.

SLEEP BOOSTERS

90. **Figs.** This fibrous fruit contains sleep-inducing tryptophan.
91. **Wild lettuce.** Leafy greens that contain the sedative lactucarium.
92. **Sesame seeds.** Their omega-6s support healthy sleep patterns.

GET ADVENTUROUS

93. **Nettles.** These have purifying properties.
94. **Physalis.** High in vitamin C.
95. **Daikon radishes.** Rich in iron.
96. **Acai berries.** Antibacterial.
97. **Papaya.** Aids digestion.
98. **Okra.** A good vegetable source of calcium.
99. **Miso paste.** Rich in phyto-oestrogens.
100. **Guavas.** High in vitamin C.

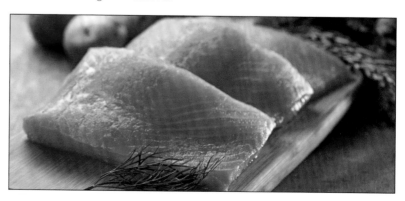

Suggested meal plan structure

Monday
Breakfast: Muesli with milk or apple juice.
Lunch: Coronation chicken sandwich on rye bread (Coronation chickpeas if vegetarian) served with creamy broccoli soup.
Dinner: Poached salmon with three different vegetables of choice. For vegetarians, vegetable stir-fry with nine vegetables, and served with rice noodles.

Tuesday
Breakfast: English muffin with steamed spinach and hollandaise sauce.
Lunch: Waldorf salad served with chicken breast, or salmon Niçoise salad.
Dinner: Moroccan Tagine with lamb, chicken or vegetables, served with rice.

Wednesday
Breakfast: Porridge or berry with a yoghurt crunch.
Lunch: Egg and cress sandwich served with side pasta salad.
Dinner: Red Thai chicken curry served with rice, vegetables and a small side salad. Butterbean Thai curry if vegetarian.

Thursday
Breakfast: Beans on wholemeal toast.
Lunch: Sweet potato minestrone soup with spelt crisp breads.
Dinner: Lamb lasagne. Layered vegetable and lentil lasagne, or root vegetable casserole if vegetarian.

Friday
Breakfast: Vegetable omelette.
Lunch: Lentil, three-bean, and vegetable soup with tuna or salmon bagel.
Dinner: Cajun Seasoned Cod with choice of three vegetables or Marinated Sea Bass with asparagus risotto. Vegetable tarts for vegetarians.

Saturday
Breakfast: Tortilla wrap with beans, scrambled egg, lettuce, and tomato.
Lunch: Baked sweet potato with various toppings (diced boiled chicken, tuna, salmon, crab, prawns) served with a side salad.
Dinner: Lamb and lentil chilli. Soya mince and lentils if vegetarian.

Sunday
Breakfast: Healthy flapjack (see www.nutrichef.co.uk for different types)
Lunch: Barley broth soup with spinach and diced lamb, chicken or extra vegetables. Served with Ryvita cracker and hummus.
Dinner: Mexican taco (build your own) with a selection of toppings, such as turkey mince, grated carrot, lettuce, tomatoes, cucumber, re-fried beans, cheese, and so on.

Some recipes

Sweet potato minestrone
1 onion (chopped)
3 celery stalks
1/2 white cabbage (thinly sliced)
2 yeast-free stock cubes
400g tin of butterbeans
2 medium-sized sweet potatoes (chopped into bite-sized chunks)
2 tbsp fresh parsley
100g macaroni pasta (cooked and cooled)

Place the onion, celery, cabbage, stock cubes, and sweet potatoes in a pan and cover with water. Bring to the boil and simmer on a lower heat for approximately 30 minutes. Add a little water if necessary. Add the butterbeans and pasta and simmer for a further 5 minutes. Divide between bowls and top with fresh parsley. Serves 6.

Asparagus risotto
115g asparagus spears
1.2 litres yeast-free vegetable stock
1 fennel bulb
1 tbsp olive oil
2 leeks (shredded)
350g Arborio rice
Pepper to taste
50g almonds (crushed to sprinkle for topping)
Optional side garnish: slices of avocado and artichokes

Blanch the asparagus and set to one side. Bring stock to the boil. In a separate pan, fry the fennel in olive oil for 3-4 minutes; add rice and fry for 2-3 minutes. Add a ladleful of stock to the pan and gently cook. Stir until absorbed and continue adding stock one ladleful at a time until the rice is tender (takes about 25 minutes). Top with pepper, asparagus, and chopped almonds.

Berry and yoghurt crunch
75g of a mix of millet flakes, barley flakes, and rice flakes
4 tbsp malt barley extract
500g dairy-free yoghurt
1 orange rind, finely grated
225g mixed berries – blueberries, blackberries, cherries

Heat a dry frying pan; add flakes and toast for 1 minute; add 2 tbsp malt extract and stir until flakes are slightly golden. Stir remaining malt extract and rind into the yoghurt. Gently add berries while stirring. To serve, layer the flakes and yoghurt, and place the berries on top. Serves 4.

Marinated sea bass in black bean sauce

Marinade:

2 fillets sea bass

3 tbsp tamari

2 tbsp maple syrup

Pepper to taste

Stir-fry:

200g beansprouts

1 finely-chopped onion

3 tbsp black bean sauce

1 head broccoli

1 tbsp sunflower oil

Marinate two fillets of sea bass in the tamari and maple syrup. Add a little pepper to taste. Marinate for 12 to 24 hours. Remove the bass from the marinade, then pan-fry until cooked through. Stir-fry the vegetables and serve with the fish on a bed of brown rice or barley.

Creamy broccoli soup

2 cups of vegetable stock or water

3-4 cups of broccoli (chopped)

1 avocado

2 onions (chopped)

1 cup of kale

1/2 cup of parsley

1 red pepper (chopped)

Cumin and ginger to taste

Gently warm the stock or water in a pan and then add the broccoli. Heat through for approximately 5 minutes. In a blender, purée the warmed broccoli with the pepper, onion, avocado, kale, and parsley. If you find this a little thick, just add a little hot water for the consistency you require. Add a little cumin and ginger to taste and serve with a slice of lemon to garnish. Serves 4-6.

Salmon Niçoise salad

1 can (400g) red salmon

400g new potatoes
  (boil until tender)

200g French beans

2 Little Gem lettuces

5 anchovies

20 cherry tomatoes (halved)

4 hard-boiled eggs

150g black olives

A sprinkle of parsley

Dressing:

1 clove of garlic (crushed)

1 tsp Dijon mustard

5 tbsp olive oil

2 tbsp balsamic vinegar

Pepper to taste

Drain the salmon; remove skin and bones; break into large chunks. Arrange lettuce in bowl; add tomatoes, potatoes, and French beans. Add anchovies, eggs, and olives. Put dressing ingredients in a jar and shake well. Drizzle over salad.

Root vegetable casserole

2 large potatoes (cubed)

4 tbsp olive oil

1 lemon (unwaxed)

1 tsp ground cumin

1 red onion (sliced thinly)

15 baby onions

4 large carrots
  (cut into chunks)

1 swede (cut into chunks)

1 tin chickpeas

1 tin chopped tomatoes

Chopped parsley
  (one handful)

2 yeast-free stock cubes

4 tbsp Flaxseed Oil (garnish only)

Fry the red onions and baby onions in oil and add the cumin and lemon. Add 225ml boiling water and melt the stock cubes. Add the rest of the ingredients and simmer for 30 minutes or until the vegetables are soft. To serve, pour a tablespoon of flaxseed oil over each portion of casserole and garnish. (Serves 4)

Bean and vegetable chilli (add lamb or minced turkey if desired)

3 tbsp olive oil

2 onions

2 cloves garlic

2 tsp mild chilli powder

2 tbsp freshly-chopped coriander

2 sticks of celery (chopped)

2 red peppers (chopped)

300ml yeast-free stock
  (kallo brand)

400g tin of chickpeas

400g tin of black-eyed peas

400g tin of chopped tomatoes

Pepper to taste

Fry the onions in olive oil until golden brown, then add the garlic, chilli powder, and pepper, and fry for 2-3 minutes. Add the peppers and celery, and fry for a further 2 minutes. Next add the stock, chickpeas, and tomatoes, and bring to the boil. Reduce the heat, cover and simmer for 20 minutes. Season again with pepper and sprinkle with fresh coriander. Serve with boiled rice.

Healthy snacks

Crudité of vegetables and salsa, hummus or guacamole, nuts and seed selections, fruit, Nutrichef flapjacks.

Andy Blow on nutrition...

In the motorsport environment, particularly at amateur level, pre-race nutrition often involves grabbing whatever is available at the paddock burger van. I am convinced that if drivers had a greater understanding of what a negative effect this is having on their performance these wagons would go out of business very quickly!

Special diets

Some diets, like liquid diets (Slimfast) and the Aitken Diet Plan are specialised. Their success rates are variable and the plans do not suit everyone. The Aitken Diet, for example, recommends a high-protein and low-carbohydrate intake. Although weight loss may occur, it may be at the expense of muscle mass rather than fat. Before starting specialised diets, seek advice from a doctor or nutrition specialist, as certain medical conditions can be worsened.

The output

Remember from the energy balance equation that reducing the input is only half of the game. To create a negative balance, energy expenditure must also be increased, and this is achieved by simply doing more exercise. Physical activity accounts for around 25% of total daily expenditure in someone like Jim, while top athletes may expend up to 80%. This wide variation means that increasing exercise is a sure way of slimming down and shedding those surplus pounds of fat.

Apart from the obvious benefits of becoming fitter, increasing physical activity pays other dividends that include:

- Less likelihood of diabetes.
- Better body functions, such as lung capacity, endurance, joint functions, etc.
- Better balance of fats in the blood (some fats are better than others).
- Better blood pressure control.
- Less chance of mild clinical depression and anxiety (both more common in obese people).
- Improved self-esteem and general well-being.

As well as being overweight, bordering on obese with a BMI of 30, Jim has a family history of heart disease. His father had a heart attack at an early age. Jim can reduce his risk by losing weight and exercising more. Unfortunately, instead of using exercise to relax, he tends to do little over weekends. This creates a reduction in energy expenditure of about 500kcal a day at weekends, which multiplied by 52 weekends in the year, results in an overall positive balance of 52,000kcal a year, or 3kg of weight gain. Over ten years he would put on 30kg, or 5 stone, in weight!

The late Colin McRae on his intake...

I watch what I eat the whole time, especially the week before an event and during the rally itself. Eat lots of different things and the right amount of everything with not too much fatty and sweet stuff. Chicken, pasta, meat, fish and salads – basically a good Mediterranean diet ...

and on his output...

I cycle, do moto-cross, jet and water skiing ... stuff that I enjoy doing otherwise it gets boring if you just jog around the block every morning.

So what exercise should I do to lose weight?

As with any exercise plan, it is recommended that you consult a doctor before starting, especially if you have not exercised for some time. This chapter is not only for those who are overweight. It should also be useful as a general guide for those who want to maintain their weight during the race season.

The recommendations of the UK Health Education Authority in 1998 were:

For improved health and to help in weight management, adults should try to build up gradually, to take half-an-hour of moderate intensity physical activity on five or more days of the week. Activities like brisk walking, cycling, swimming, dancing, and gardening are good options!

Stick to the following recommendations and you should lose weight:

- Exercise intensity should be to a level where you can just about talk without getting out of breath. Your breathing, however, should be slightly harder than normal.
- Go for 30 minutes of activity every day, even if it means three 10-minute periods or two 15-minute periods accumulated throughout the day.

- Consider going for longer sessions of up to 45 minutes to really shed the fat. This extended period of exercise uses fat as a preferential energy source and is also known as the 'slow-burn' by some.
- If you have a heart-rate monitor, go for an intensity that keeps your heart rate at about 60% of maximum. If you are generally unfit you will be surprised at how low an intensity exercise is needed to reach this!
- Go for exercises that use the large muscles of the body and are aerobic (get you breathing hard and increase your heart rate). These include cycling, running, and swimming.

Jim decides to make lifestyle changes. He continues to eat the same, but increases his output by walking to work every day. This takes 20 minutes each way and at a leisurely pace burns 180kcal a day in total. At the weekends he decides to take up swimming for 30 minutes each day. Over three months he will burn 14,400kcal, or the equivalent of 1.6kg (3.5lb) of fat. All this without even modifying his input!

The table in *Fig. 3* shows the calories spent doing common activities over one hour for an average 70kg (11 stone) man. Remember that if you are heavier you will burn more calories.

How much should I aim to lose?

For best results, weight loss should be gradual rather than sudden. That way, instead of fighting it, the body gets a chance to adjust to the loss.

Assuming you adjust your input and increase your output accordingly, and stick to this change, you can lose up to 2kg (4-5lb) in the first week. This is because most of the initial loss is owing to glycogen (a form of carbohydrate) breaking down, and this requires a lot of water. Weight loss will slow down after this as fat begins to break down. This is not an indication that your plans have failed, so do not give up! If you lose around 0.5-1kg per week after the initial drop you will be doing well!

Key body systems
Immune system

The immune system protects the body from potentially harmful substances. The inflammatory response (inflammation) is part of innate immunity. It occurs when tissues are injured by bacteria, trauma, toxins, heat, or any other cause.

Tips to boost the immune system
- **Lemon** is the ideal food for restoring the acid-alkaline balance of the body. Drinking freshly squeezed lemon juice in water, or adding it to tea, salad dressings (in place of vinegar), baking or cooking, helps maintain the body's internal 'climate' at a pH which supports healthy bacteria instead of the viruses and harmful bacteria which thrive in more acidic

Activity	kcal per hour	Activity	kcal per hour
Aerobics	420	Soccer	480
Brisk walking	305	Stair climbing	630
Brushing teeth	175	Swimming	620
Gardening	335	Strolling leisurely	220
Jogging	695	Washing the car	315
Mowing the lawn	335	Watching TV	75
Playing cards	120	Weight lifting	215
Shovelling snow	415	Working at the gym	400

ABOVE: Fig. 3. The calories burnt doing everyday work. *(Taken with permission from Calorie Control Council, www.caloriecontrol.org)*

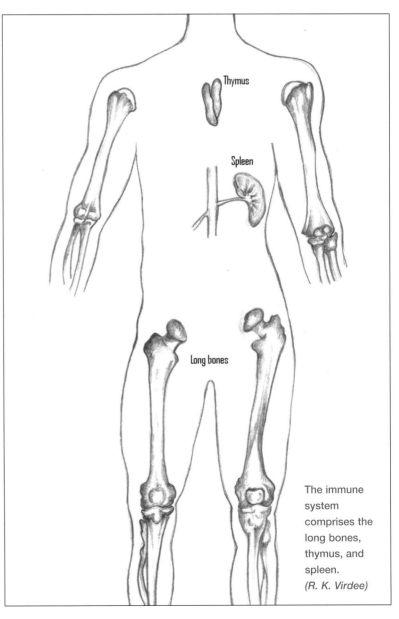

Thymus

Spleen

Long bones

The immune system comprises the long bones, thymus, and spleen.
(R. K. Virdee)

environments. Cider apple vinegar is another great way to improve your body's alkalinity, but the taste of lemons is much more pleasant!

■ **Good quality protein.** Protein is a building block for a healthy body, mind, and immune system. A diet low in protein tends to be high in carbohydrates which convert readily to glucose, spiking blood sugar levels and stressing the pancreas and the immune system.

■ **Stop drinking coffee.** Contrary to recent marketing as a source of antioxidants, chocolate and coffee are two of the worst things you can consume for your immune system and your health. Caffeine robs your body of minerals and vitamins, and it dehydrates you. If you drink coffee, make sure you add an additional two glasses to your water intake per cup of coffee. A mineral supplement helps to offset caffeine's damage, too.

■ **Drink plenty of water.** Most headaches occur because of dehydration. Despite the number of reminders, people still aren't getting enough water! Headaches and thirst are both signs of dehydration. You should be drinking, in daily ounces, half your body weight in pounds – i.e. body weight in pounds, divided by 2 = number of ounces of water per day.

■ **Cut out sugar.** If you do only one thing to boost your immune system, then you won't do better than eliminating sugar. You will see noticeable results in your energy levels, weight

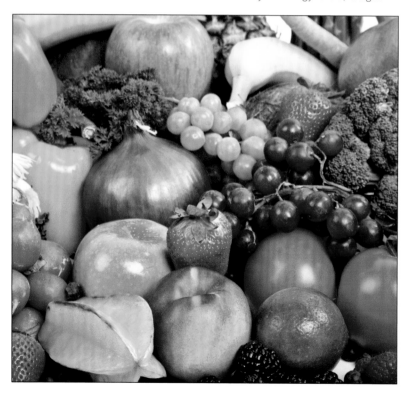

distribution, immunity, and your ability to think clearly when you break the cravings and stop eating refined sugar. Many holistic nutritionists consider sugar an adverse drug for its impact on the human body. Sugar alternatives, such as agave and stevia, do exist, but avoid artificial sweeteners as they are more toxic than cane sugar.

■ **Stock up on raw fruits and vegetables for their antioxidants, vitamins, minerals, fibre and enzymes.** The nutritional content that you receive from raw fruits and vegetables is unparalleled. Many vitamins, including C, are antioxidants and will protect cells – including those of your immune system – from damage by toxins in the environment. Dark-coloured produce (berries, kale, and broccoli) tends to be higher in flavonoids, polyphenols, and other antioxidants. The perfect source of minerals is seaweed, which is sold dried, but can often be found raw (dried at low temperatures to maintain most of the enzymes and nutrients), in health food stores.

Foods to boost the immune system

■ **Citrus fruit**
Oranges and grapefruit are all packed with protective nutrients such as vitamin C and bioflavonoids that help to ward off winter colds and flu.

■ **The pumpkin family**
Butternut, pumpkin, and squash are all great sources of beta-carotene – one of the most powerful antioxidants.

■ **Probiotic foods**
By now, you've probably heard that probiotic supplements and foods, like yoghurt and tempeh (a dish made from split soybeans and water), are good for you.

■ **Fish**
Fish is a fantastic, healthy and versatile source of zinc and the omega-3 fatty acids.

■ **Garlic**
Garlic does more than add flavour to your food. This pungent vegetable also has antibacterial and antiviral effects, and seems to be particularly useful in combating chest infections.

■ **Mushrooms**
Recent studies have found that certain mushrooms are good for the immune system. The varieties known as Reishi, Maitake, and Shiitake seem to be particularly useful.

■ **Oats**
A great source of carbohydrates, protein, vitamins, and minerals. Their low GI means they stabilise blood-sugar levels and help keep you sustained for longer.

Digestive system

The digestive system prepares food for use by hundreds of millions of body cells. Food when eaten cannot reach cells (because it cannot pass through the intestinal walls to the bloodstream. The gut modifies food physically and chemically and disposes of unusable waste. Physical and chemical modification (digestion) depends on exocrine and endocrine secretions and controlled movement of food through the digestive tract.

Digestive complaints: bloating and wind; indigestion after meals; stomach cramps; heartburn, stomach ulcers, acid reflux.

Foods to eliminate:

- **Dairy products** (including milk, cheese, and butter)
- **Eggs**
- **Wheat** (in bread and cereals)
- **Coffee and caffeinated beverages** (i.e. tea, fizzy drinks, and chocolate)
- **Alcohol**

Foods to eat:

- **Pineapples** – contain an enzyme called bromelain, which aids digestion.
- **Artichokes** – aid digestion and stabilise blood sugar, two important factors for weight loss. They also lower cholesterol and help protect against liver disease.
- **Papaya** – contains an enzyme called papain, which aids digestion.
- **Lemons** – help keep the correct acid/alkaline balance of the body.
- **Cider apple vinegar** – alkalising to the body and helps keep the correct acid/alkaline balance of the body.
- **Root vegetables** – (radish, carrots, fennel, and parsley root). All contain fibre, vitamins, and minerals, along with enzymes for proper digestion.
- **Figs** – are beneficial for constipation, digestion, and anaemia. They help protect against cancer.
- **Beansprouts** – are rich in digestible energy, bioavailable vitamins, minerals, amino acids, proteins, beneficial enzymes, and phytochemicals.
- **Licorice** – relaxes muscles and can help alleviate stomach cramps.
- **Ginger** – has a calming and soothing effect on the digestive system.

Endocrine/glandular system

The endocrine/glandular system is a communication network that regulates basic drives and emotions, promotes growth and sexual identity, assists in the repair of broken tissue,

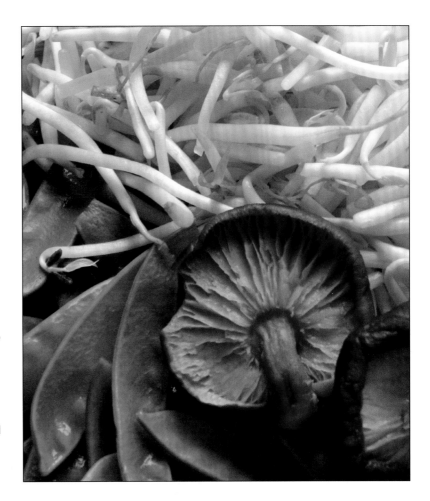

and helps generate energy. The ductless glands secrete substances which are released directly into the circulation and which influence metabolism and other body functions.

Common concerns: menstrual problems; PMT; menopausal concerns; hormone imbalances; loss of libido; prostate problems; diabetes.

Foods to avoid:

- **Sweets and Sugars.** Sugar causes an imbalance to the hormonal system and will lead to adrenal exhaustion.
- **Refined starches.** White bread, pasta, cereals, and pastries should all be avoided.
- **Limit meat and animal protein.** The high fat content of high protein diets can upset the glandular system.
- **Nicotine, alcohol and tobacco** products cause swings in blood-sugar levels and stimulate the production of adrenaline.
- **Avoid hidden sugars:** see list!
- **Avoid sweeteners** – sorbitol, aspartame, hexanol, mannitol, and glycol.
- **Avoid salt** – it exhausts the adrenals and causes a loss of potassium, leading to lower blood-sugar.

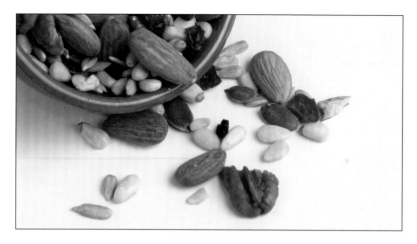

Foods to eat:
- Plenty of Fruits and Vegetables
- Eat a high-fibre diet and vegetables that are raw or steamed
- Beans and legumes
- Lentils
- Brown rice
- Potatoes
- Soy products
- Apricots
- Apples – high pectin
- Bananas
- Grapefruit
- Lemons
- Melons
- Licorice – helps stabilise blood sugar and nourishes the adrenal glands
- Bilberries and wild yams – help control insulin levels
- Spirulina – helps to stabilise blood sugar and rich in vitamin B12
- Almonds
- Fruit smoothies

Nervous system

The brain and nervous system are probably the most complex and sensitive physiological structures in the human body. The importance of a healthy diet in the maintenance of these structures should not be underestimated. The complex effect of nutrition on brain function and the health of the central nervous system is often a neglected field, and most people do not associate the foods they eat with the psychological conditions they develop.

In this section, we take a look at several important issues.

Minerals and your nervous system

While it is important for us to have a balanced diet that supplies all the necessary minerals to keep our bodies functioning at an optimum level, certain minerals – such as iron and iodine – are vital at certain stages of our development to ensure that our brains and nervous systems develop normally.

Iron
Iron is a mineral that is used to produce healthy haemoglobin (a biological pigment contained in the red blood cells) that is capable of transporting oxygen to the entire body. All our cells require oxygen to survive, but the brain is the most sensitive organ in the body when it comes to oxygen deprivation.

Food sources of iron:
- Lentils
- Red meat (beef, mutton, pork, and venison)
- Poultry
- Fish
- Parsley
- Iron-fortified breakfast cereals
- Molasses
- Sesame seeds
- Green leafy vegetables
- Dried fruit
- Spinach

Iodine
Iodine is the main component of the hormone thyroxine. This hormone influences our metabolic rate; in other words, the speed at which all body processes occur.

Food sources of iodine:
- Seafood
- Fish
- Leafy green vegetables
- Kelp
- Seaweeds/spirulina
- Garlic

B-vitamins
Foods rich in B-vitamins are important for the brain and nervous system. Brain chemicals are synthesised from amino acids and require B-vitamins for their production. Food sources of vitamin B include avocados, bean sprouts, bananas, green leafy vegetables, nuts, soya products, and yeast extract.

Structural system

The structural system, like a building frame, helps our body withstand stresses and strains. This system also houses all the other systems of the body and protects them from the outside environment. It consists of bones, muscles, and connective tissue.

Calcium depletion

Women, especially as they grow older, are far more prone to suffer from the increasing fragility of their structural systems, but no one is immune. Diet and lifestyle play a major role in determining who is at risk. Some foods, habits, and even medications can be immensely harmful to the bones and connective tissues. For example, alcohol may cause loss of bone mass. Animal studies indicate that high doses of alcohol inhibit calcium absorption and may even be toxic to bone cells. Likewise, smoking is bad because it depletes the vitamin C needed for proper production of collagen, a cementing substance that holds body cells together. A few prescription drugs – such as cortisone, some anti-convulsants, and thyroid medications – present a possible risk. Even caffeine, in large enough amounts, can cause a significant loss of calcium, as can aspirin and mineral oil – including the mineral oil found in some cosmetics, which can penetrate the skin and end up in the bloodstream.

Common concerns: arthritis; dermatitis; warts; cold sores; skin conditions; osteoporosis; muscle cramps.

Foods to avoid:
- Dairy products (including milk, cheese, and eggs)
- Wheat (including bread and cereals)
- Salt and processed foods
- White and refined flour (including bread, pasta and pastries)
- Caffeine
- Alcohol and cigarettes

Foods to Include:
- Broccoli
- Spring greens, leafy vegetables
- Kale
- Almonds
- Tofu
- Calcium-fortified dairy-free milk (i.e. rice, oat, almond, soya and quinoa milk.)
- Nuts and seeds
- Canned fish (including salmon and sardines)
- Beans and legumes
- Whole grains

Urinary system

The urinary system keeps the chemicals and water in balance by removing a type of waste, called urea, from the blood. Urea is produced when foods containing protein, such as meat, poultry, and certain vegetables, are broken down in the body. Urea is carried in the bloodstream to the kidneys.

Common concerns: bladder/kidney infection; kidney stones; incontinence; cystitis; diabetes; kidney cysts; water retention and back pain.

Tips for a healthy urinary system
- Drink plenty of fluids (ideally water) to keep your urine volume at or above two litres a day. This may mean drinking up to three litres of fluid a day, including drinking at night, especially when exercising regularly. Drinking fluids can halve your risk of getting a second stone by lowering concentrations of stone-forming chemicals.
- Avoid drinking too much tea or coffee.
- Citrus juices (particularly orange, grapefruit, and cranberry) may reduce the risk of some stones. Mineral water cannot cause kidney stones because it contains only trace elements of minerals.
- Reducing salt intake may lower the risk of calcium-based stones.
- Avoid very high and very low calcium intake. A low calcium diet may in fact be associated with an increased rate of recurrent stones.
- Don't drink more than one litre each week of drinks with phosphoric acid, which is used to flavour carbonated drinks such as cola and beer.

Foods to eat:
- Plenty of fresh fruits and vegetables
- Cranberries and cranberry juice
- Raisins
- Bananas – rich in potassium
- Red fruits/berries/grapes
- Water melon
- Tomatoes – contain lycopene, beneficial to the urinary tract
- Grapefruits
- Peaches

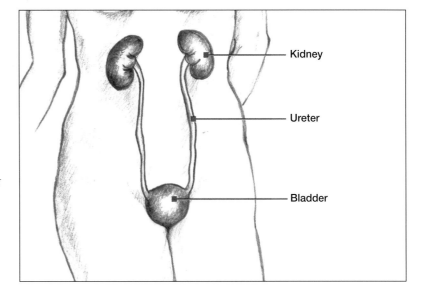

BELOW: The urinary system filters blood with the kidneys and transports urine to the bladder via the ureters. *(R. K. Virdee)*

Kidney

Ureter

Bladder

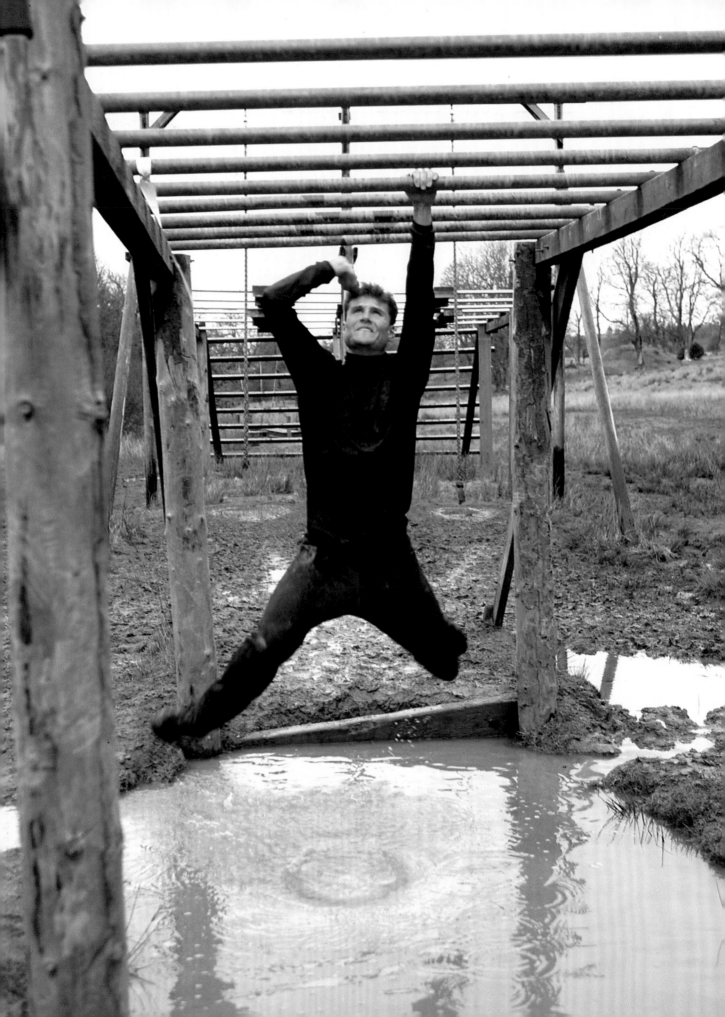

10

Motorsport-specific circuit training

Circuit training is a superb method of conditioning for motor racers. It develops strength, cardiovascular conditioning, reaction/agility skills, and mental toughness, as it can be very intensive. It is also a very efficient way to train, as you can squeeze a great workout into 30-50 minutes with limited equipment and space.

A typical circuit involves 8 to 12 exercises and follows a structure that includes exercises to work the upper body, lower body, trunk/core, and improve reaction/agility skills. It is the reaction and agility work that makes it very specific to the

demands of racing, teaching you to think and move with great pace and precision when under high levels of physical pressure. When doing circuit training, the emphasis is on fast movements and high numbers of reps to get your heart rate up, as well as working the specific muscles involved in each exercise. In other words, there is no loafing around – it's all GO, GO, GO once the circuit is underway!

Use the circuits outlined here as a basis to design your own routines. Don't feel that you are limited to only the exercises listed below.

OPPOSITE: David Coulthard on a training session that would help him develop all the different components of fitness. *(Mike Gibon, MVG Photographic)*

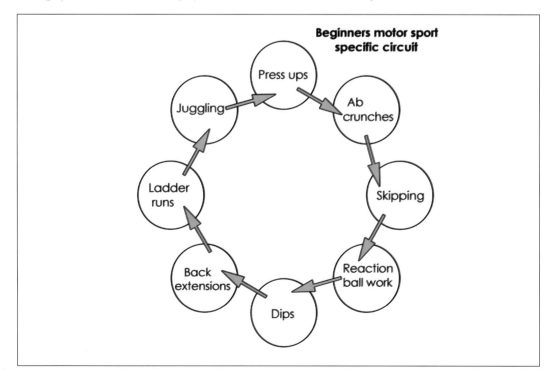

Beginners motor sport specific circuit

Press ups — Ab crunches — Skipping — Reaction ball work — Dips — Back extensions — Ladder runs — Juggling — Press ups

LEFT: Organisation of a motorsport-specific circuit for beginners.

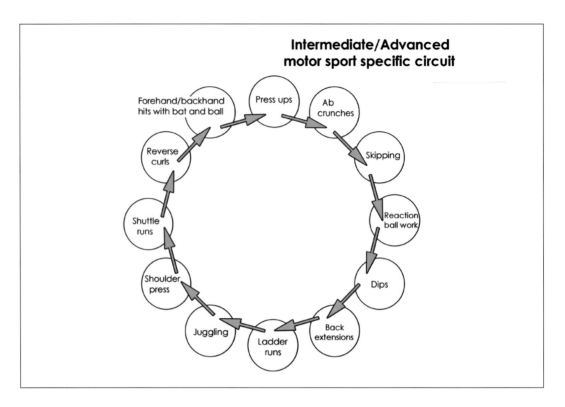

RIGHT: Organisation of a motorsport-specific circuit for intermediate/advanced drivers.

Intermediate/Advanced motor sport specific circuit

Be creative, bearing in mind the following considerations.

1   The exercises follow the order:
- Upper body
- Trunk
- Lower body
- Agility/reaction

This stops any one body part being overloaded excessively and ensures a balanced routine for the whole body.

2   Exercises need to be done fast and repetitively, so choose those that do not require a high level of complex technique or fiddly equipment to perform.

3   Perform each exercise for a set amount of time, starting with 30 seconds, and allow yourself 30 seconds to move to the next station. Two to three sets of eight exercises is a good place to begin. You can gradually increase the amount of stations to around 12, then the number of sets to four or five, and finally the length of time on each station towards 60 seconds as you improve.

4   Count the number of reps that you achieve on each exercise and aim to match or beat it in the following set.

5   A good warm up and substantial cool down before and after the main part of the session are essential.

Two to three circuits per week during the off season is a realistic reflection of the amount of sessions needed to stimulate improvement. If you build up the intensity and length of the sessions to peak just before the season begins, you can then revert to just one circuit per week when racing regularly. This will then be sufficient to maintain the fitness and form you have created, without risking fatigue and stiffness going into competitions – especially important if you have a busy competitive

Example lists of exercises to build up your own circuits

Upper body
- Press ups
- Shoulder press
- Bicep curls
- Dips
- Boxing

Lower body
- Ladder runs
- Hexagon jumps
- Shuttle runs
- Skipping

Ab and trunk
- Crunches
- Back extensions
- Reverse curls
- Plank variations

Reaction/skill
- Reaction ball
- Juggling
- Throwing and catching (one leg and knee bent, with partner or against a wall)
- Forehand/backhand keep-ups with bat and ball

schedule. Change the exercises round on a regular basis to broaden your fitness base and avoid overuse injuries. Training with a partner on these sets can be very motivating if you time each other and try to compete on the number of reps completed on each set.

Example beginners circuit

All eight exercises 30 seconds work with 30 seconds recovery to move to the next station. Repeat the circuit three times with a five-minute break between sets.
- Press-ups
- Ab crunches
- Skipping
- Reaction ball work
- Dips
- Back extensions
- Ladder runs
- Juggling

Example intermediate circuit

All 12 exercises 30 seconds work with 30 seconds recovery to move to the next station. Repeat the circuit three times with a five-minute break between sets.
- Press-ups
- Ab crunches
- Skipping
- Reaction ball work
- Dips

- Back extensions
- Ladder runs
- Juggling
- Shoulder press
- Shuttle runs
- Reverse curls
- Forehand/backhand hits with bat and ball

Example advanced circuit

All 12 exercises of the intermediate circuit, but with 45 seconds work and 15 seconds recovery to move to the next station. Repeat the circuit three times with a five-minute break between sets.

Circuit training is one of the most potent forms of training available to racing drivers. If you ever find yourself in a situation where training time is limited, a quick dose of circuits two or three times per week is one of the best methods to maintain all-round fitness until you can resume a full programme of activity.

Andy Blow on circuit training with Renault F1 drivers...

When I was working with Bernie Shrosbree at Renault F1 we often did circuit sessions with all three drivers (two race drivers and the test driver) at the same time. At every station you could see the guys counting the reps and trying to beat each other. The level of intensity that this created really pushed their performance to new levels every time.

BELOW: Regular group training sessions both indoors and outside were key to the physical training at Renault F1. (Renault F1)

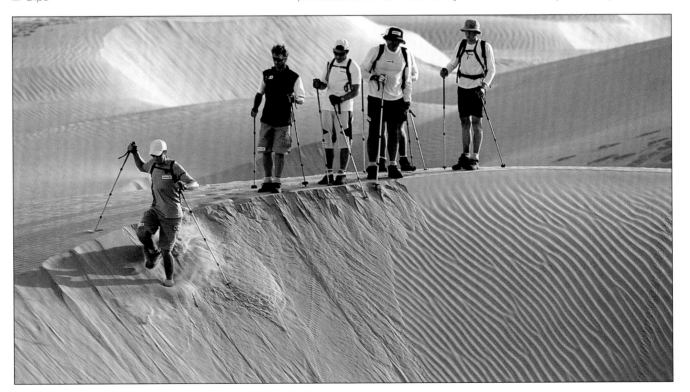

The following sequences show examples of exercises that can be easily incorporated into a motorsport-specific circuit. Each works on a different part of the body as well as developing reaction times. *(Dave Blow, myeyefor)*

RIGHT AND FAR RIGHT: Bench jumps (agility and stamina).

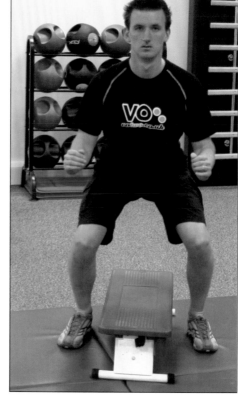 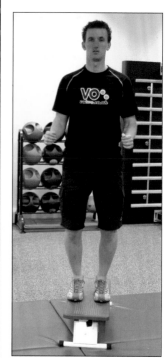

BELOW (LEFT & RIGHT): Biceps (strength).

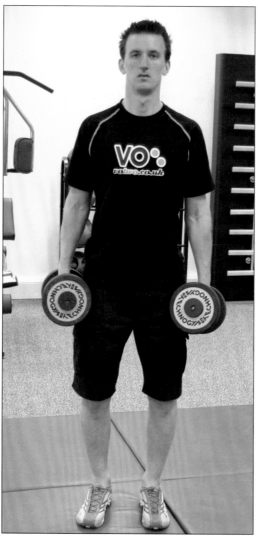 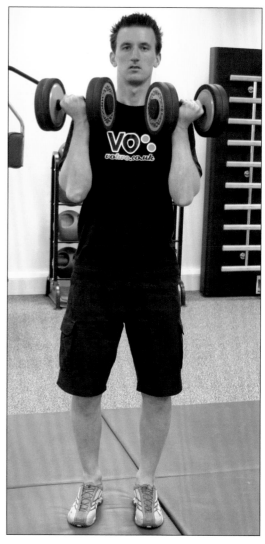

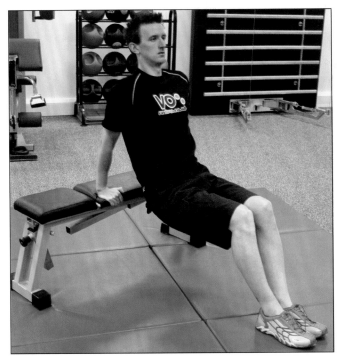
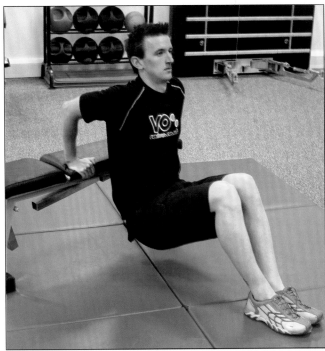

ABOVE (LEFT & RIGHT): Dips (strength).

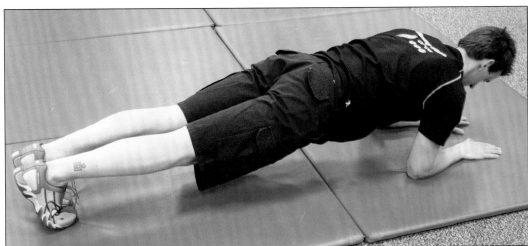

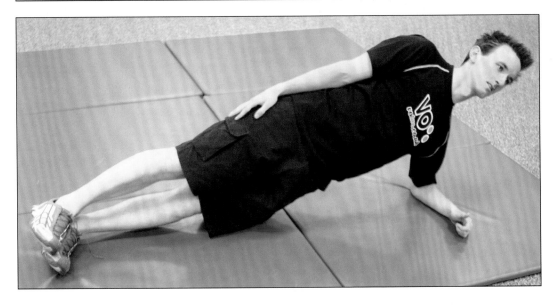

CENTRE AND LEFT: Plank – side and front (core strength).

RIGHT AND INSET: Ladder (speed and agility).

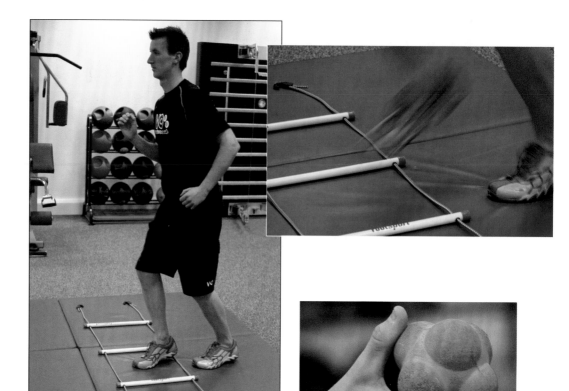

BELOW AND INSET: Reaction Z-ball (reaction and co-ordination).

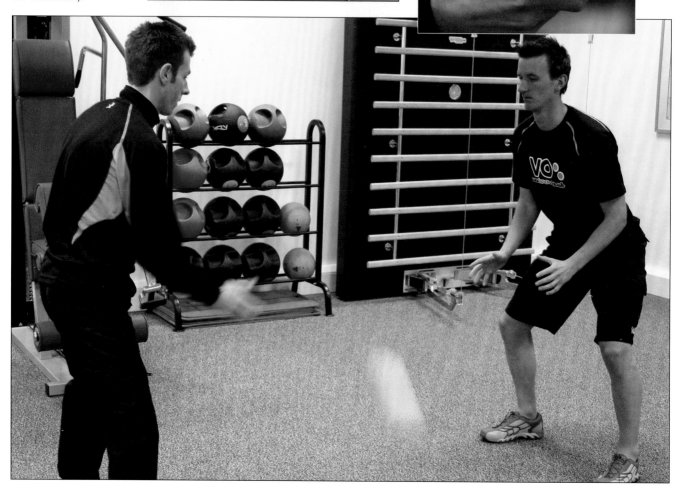

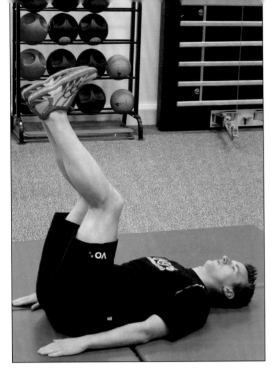 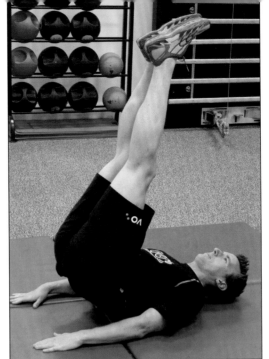

LEFT AND BELOW:
Reverse curl, with or
without Swiss ball (core
strength).

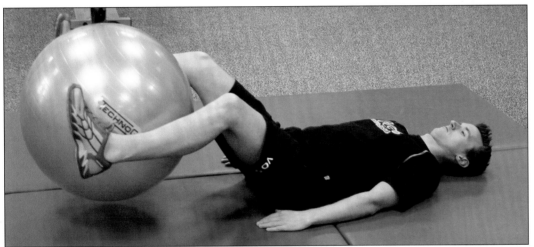

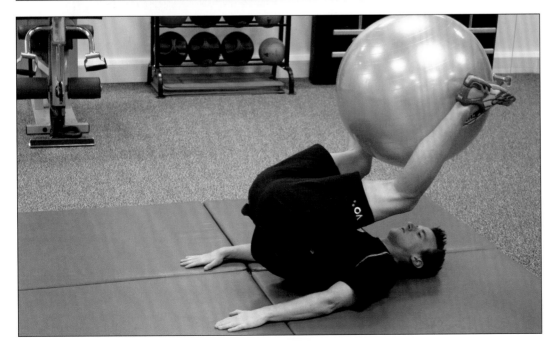

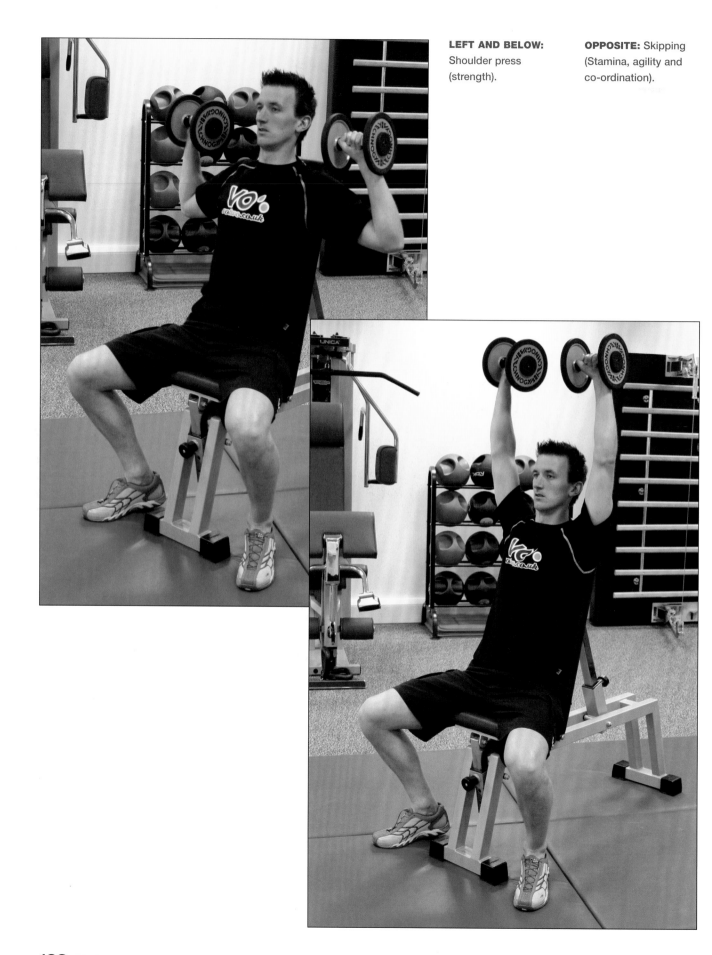

LEFT AND BELOW: Shoulder press (strength).

OPPOSITE: Skipping (Stamina, agility and co-ordination).

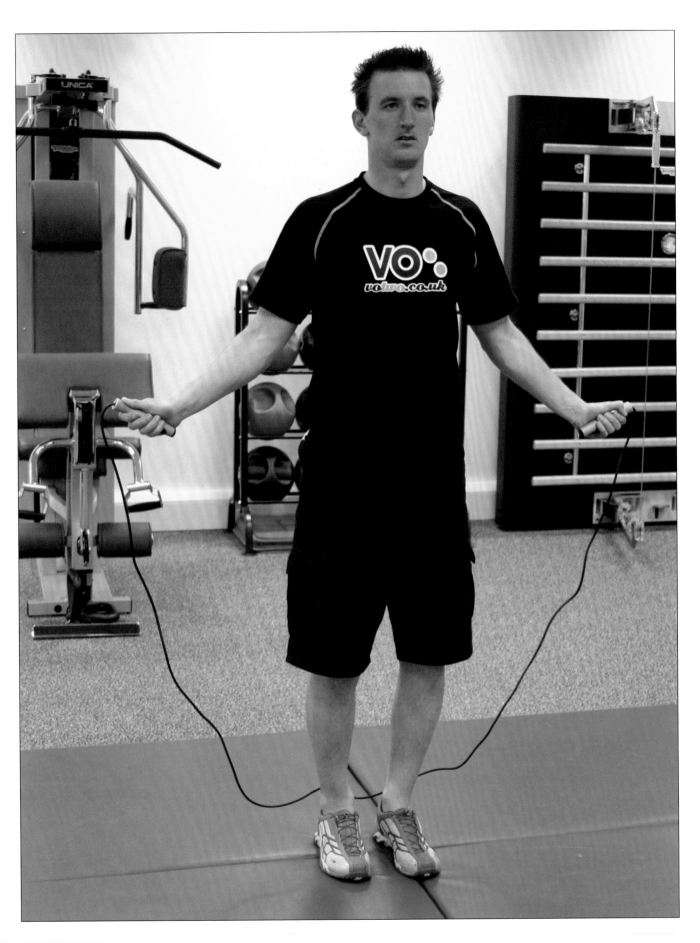

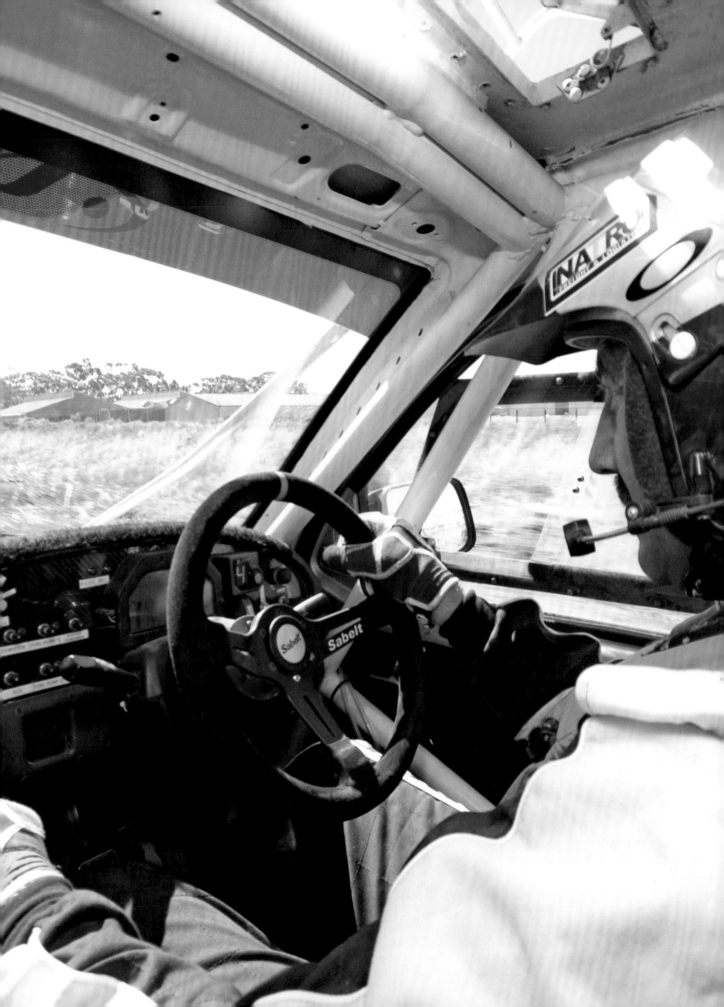

11

The event

This chapter gives you guidelines on what to do and what to avoid during the days leading up to an event. The advice is based on scientific and medical principles currently applied by many athletes, and there is no reason why these principles cannot be adopted by motorsport competitors to give them the racing edge on the day. There are many types of motorsport events ranging from short sprints, such as drag racing, to ultra-marathons, like the Paris-Dakar rally lasting over 20 days, but whilst competitor requirements will vary from event to event, the basic principles remain the same.

Andy Blow on race day routine…
Elite athletes and drivers are always very good at maximising their performance on the day, whatever the circumstances and conditions. They have an armoury of routines and strategies to cope with whatever the event throws at them, and as a result perform to the best of their ability more regularly than their competitors.

Training
In the week of the event, training intensity should be reduced gradually, and only a light session consisting largely of warm-up routines is recommended on the day before the event. This may be an option for professional drivers with teams responsible for race preparation. With amateurs, however, the day before the race is usually hectic and stressful. Although you may not think so, a visit to the gym may just be the thing to relax. Do try to fit in a light session or a slow jog the day before the race if at all possible.

It will probably do little for you physically, but do not underestimate the psychology. Many drivers will spend 30 minutes stretching at the gym with background music, followed by a sauna to help with visualisation and relaxation.

Meals
Dietary manipulation is a recognised method of maximising performance; even the ancient Olympians recognised this. The general consensus is that you should try to load up on carbohydrates in the days before the event. This will increase the glycogen levels in your muscles. Glycogen is what the body prefers to use during exercise, and it is the depletion of this important carbohydrate that causes fatigue. The capacity of muscle to store glycogen increases with training, so by loading up before the event you decrease the chances of fatigue during the race. Carbohydrate-loading should ideally start in the week before the event. Examples of carbohydrate-rich food are rice, pasta, noodles, and potatoes.

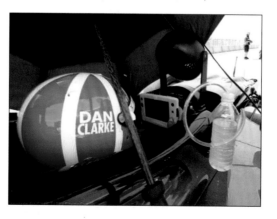

OPPOSITE: Heat production during motor racing. The competitor generates heat by muscular work. Conduction from the engine, the closed cockpit environment, and race overalls all increase the body temperature and rate of sweating. *(Kolesky/ SanDisk/Red Bull Photofiles)*

LEFT: In 1982 the Medical Commission for FISA issued guidelines for fluid intake in Formula 1 racing. It was recommended that drivers should drink 5 litres on race day. Dan Clarke, World Series Champ Car driver, complies. *(Michael Levitt, LAT USA Photography 2007)*

RIGHT: Assessing urine colour is a good method of evaluating hydration status and has been used by many national teams, such as the England cricket squad during tours in hot countries. Competitors should aim for pale straw-coloured urine. Reprinted, with permission, from L. E. Armstrong, 2000. 'Performing in extreme environments' *(Champaign, IL: Human Kinetics)*

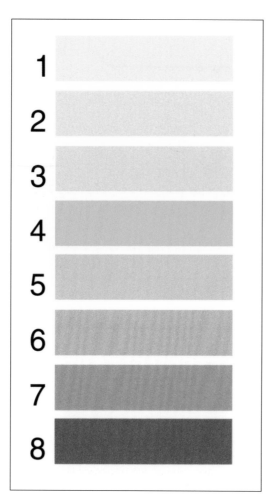

The 72 hours before an event are particularly important for maximising muscle levels of glycogen, so aim for up to 70-80% of total intake from your meals to be carbohydrates if you can. Increasing glycogen levels is of special fatigue prevention benefit with endurance races lasting typically more than 1-1½ hours, but even with shorter events stores must be maximised, especially if there is little chance of topping up levels during the day of the event. Beware, though, that glycogen-loading may cause a temporary weight gain of around 1kg (2½lb) as extra water is needed to store it.

Hydration

It is much easier to hydrate fully in the 72 hour run-up to the event than to leave it to the night before, and it would be a major mistake to start an event in a dehydrated state. If you were to do so you would risk heat exhaustion, especially in the close confines of a cockpit and wearing a three-layer fireproof suit. In the WRC Safari Rally, cockpit temperatures may be as high as 55°C, and if you start the race behind in fluid intake it is highly unlikely you will be able to make up the deficit, considering you may lose as much as a litre for every hour you sit in the car. With only around four service stops per leg, lasting around 20 minutes each, it means you have to drink almost constantly.

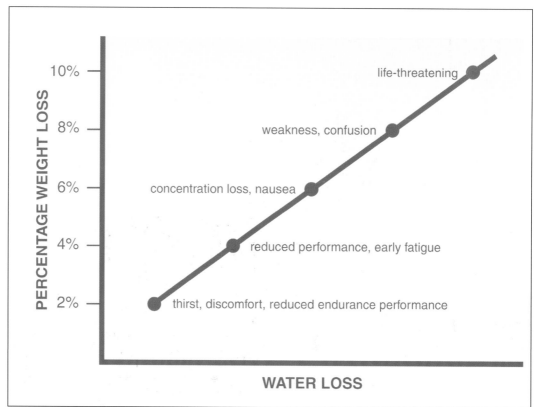

RIGHT: The relationship between dehydration and human performance.

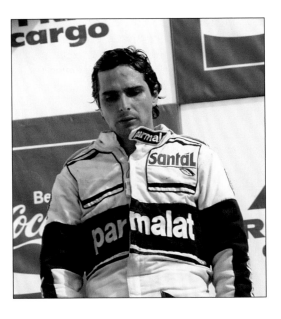

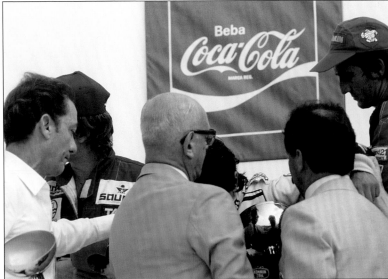

If you are dehydrated you will produce urine less frequently and in smaller quantities, as the body conserves all the water it can. The colour of the urine also tends to be darker and it may have a strong smell to it. You should learn to recognise your hydration status from your urine colour and from what your body tells you, i.e. your symptoms. Use a urine colour chart to maintain a reasonable hydration level. The symptoms of early dehydration include fatigue and headache. Increase your fluid intake if these symptoms are present.

Hyponatraemia

In recent years the problem of athletes (particularly those competing in long endurance events in the heat) over-drinking water whilst trying to avoid dehydration has become more prevalent. It is possible that this is partly due to an increased awareness of the need to hydrate fully, but a corresponding lack of knowledge about the pitfalls of overdoing it. If you drink too much water it can adversely affect the body's electrolyte balance, most significantly reducing the concentration of

ABOVE (LEFT & RIGHT): The podium collapse from dehydration. This incident, involving Nelson Piquet, led to the development of guidelines on fluid intake. *(Mike Gibbon, MVG Photographic)*

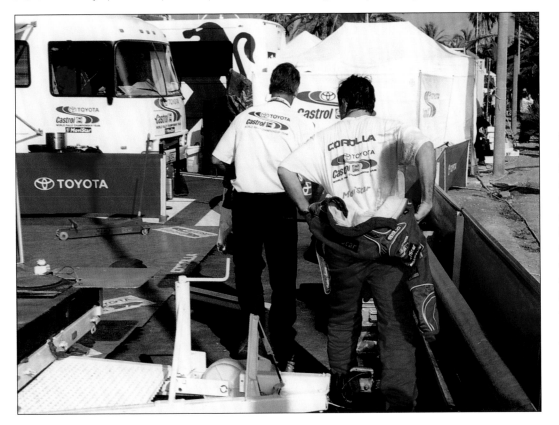

LEFT: Some rounds of the World Rally Championship are notorious for their high temperatures. FIA-regulation three-layer fireproof race suits can act as a barrier to sweat loss that can exceed a litre for every hour in the car. The competitor seen here has lost so much sweat that the dye from his race suit has come off on to his T-shirt. *(Maurice Selden, Martin Holmes Rallying)*

sodium in the bloodstream. Appropriate sodium balance is crucial for various bodily functions, and symptoms such as vomiting, nausea, cramps, and headaches can occur if it is not maintained. In severe cases, untreated hyponatraemia can lead to coma and death, so understanding how to avoid the condition is critical. It tends to occur in the heat as high sweat losses cause sodium to be lost from the body (in the form of salt that you will often see on overalls and helmet straps after a hot race). If the only fluids that are used to replace sweat contain no sodium, then it is possible that the relative concentrations in the body start to fall. The best way to avoid hyponatraemia is, therefore, to use sports drinks with added sodium. If necessary, take in some extra salt with meals and drink to match sweat losses, but try not to exceed them massively. If you start to feel bloated, unwell, and are urinating high volumes of very clear liquid, reduce your fluid intake until the symptoms recede, and seek medical attention immediately. Read on to see how to make your own sports drinks with the right amount of salt.

What you drink will depend on what you do in the days leading up to the event. If you are training, then a sports drink with carbohydrate content may be needed to provide energy as well as fluid. Otherwise, plenty of water, flavoured or not, should be sufficient. Drinking regular soft drinks will give you a large calorie boost that you may not need. They may also contain caffeine that will dehydrate you. Because of this it is advisable to avoid coffee and soft drinks in the 72 hours before the event. Remember, too, that alcohol is a potent dehydrator!

The late Colin McRae MBE ...

I don't drink alcohol at all during the recce, and if I know that an event is going to be particularly tough I won't drink at all in the week before I leave. This can be particularly tough when all your mates are off down to the pub and going out, but it's really important to keep hydrated and in training.

Iain McPherson, Supersport biker ...

During a race weekend it is important also to relax, either by watching a video or television in the motorhome, or by going to the swimming pool for a swim and a sauna and jacuzzi.

The night before the event

This is undoubtedly a crucial time for all competitors, but instead of paying attention to maximising performance potential for the event

the next morning, many amateur competitors are found in the bar, until quite late, catching up with old friends. It's something they'll probably regret in the cold light of day.

It is best to avoid alcohol altogether. Should you have a drink, try to drink water before going to bed. There is a clear relationship between human performance and hydration status. Dehydration of as little as 2% of body weight (1.4kg or 1,400ml in a 70kg competitor) will cause you to feel thirsty and uncomfortable, and it will reduce your performance in endurance events. Up to 4% water loss (2.8kg or 2,800ml in a 70kg competitor) will reduce performance, lower urine output and lead to early fatigue. You may also experience nausea and vomiting. A 5% loss has been shown to reduce aerobic capacity by 30%. A loss of up to 6% (4.2kg or 4,200ml in a 70kg competitor) will affect concentration. Losses beyond this are dangerous as they cause physical weakness and confusion. In 1982 the Medical Commission for FISA issued guidelines for fluid intake in Formula 1 racing. This followed Nelson Piquet's podium collapse from dehydration after his win at the Brazilian Grand Prix the same year. It was recommended that drivers should drink 5 litres on race day. Do bear in mind, however, that this is based on F1 races lasting 90min or more, often in very hot climates, so some common sense needs to be applied if your races are shorter or in a much milder environment.

Sleep

Top athletes routinely retire to bed early the night before an event. Not only do they gain valuable rest, they also make time to prepare themselves mentally using techniques such as some of those described in Chapter 7. However, in amateur motorsport, adequate sleep is sometimes difficult with the stress of the approaching event, especially for those competitors who also double up as the main organiser of their racing team. Don't underestimate the value of a good night's sleep, and try your level best to get at least 8-10 hours of quality shut-eye. Very often the night two nights before the event is the most critical as you can operate reasonably effectively with one night of bad sleep, but two in a row is more detrimental.

Iain McPherson, Supersport biker ...

My training intensity and quality three days before the race is restricted to a light run round the circuit. No exercise is taken the night before, and on the morning of the race a light stretch is undertaken. As for the meal content, from three days before to the morning of the event my diet consists generally of pasta, bread, and bananas, or foods of similar nature. I keep myself hydrated at all times, taking energy drinks before and during practice runs. I also try to keep a constant sleep pattern over race weekends – in bed by 9.30pm and lights out by 10pm.

Psychology

Many competitors find imagery (visualisation) particularly useful the night before the event, but don't do it just before trying to sleep as it can bring about emotions similar to those during the race. By this time most competitors will be familiar with the race circuit or have an idea of the stages involved and this, of course, helps the visualisation. The night before a race is also a good time to set some targets, taking into account the starting order and the opposition, and also to practise some positive self-talk. Any anxiety can be countered by progressive muscle relaxation.

Louise Aitken-Walker MBE ...
I'd go to bed fairly early. I shut myself in my room and watch telly, read a book, and completely chill out. I had to keep myself as calm as I could be.

Iain McPherson, Supersport biker ...
It is good to feel a bit of pressure before a race. It shows that you are switched on. You should be focusing only on the race, and entering the race confident that you've trained hard, and that you are confident in your abilities. Nothing else should enter your mind. I sometimes tell myself that this will be the last day I live, so I can push myself to the limit.

Bernie Shrosbree recommends ...
The night before a race it is a good idea to eat a light meal fairly early, maybe perform some light mobility work or easy cardiovascular training (e.g. a brisk walk) to aid relaxation and focus. If available, a massage can be of benefit, or a swim if facilities allow.

The morning of the event

This is probably the most anxious time for most! Each one has their own way of coping with pre-competition nerves, so whatever works for you, stick with it!

Always rise early, at least three hours before the event starts. Getting dressed should be at a leisurely pace. Aim to be at the event venue at least 1 to 1½ hours before the start. En route to the venue use any aids that work for you. Some like to keep quiet and focused, while others recommend listening to music. Whatever your routine, try to keep it specific every time you race so it optimises your arousal. Specific routines have been shown to improve consistency of results.

Pre-event meal

Do not compete on an empty stomach, otherwise you risk fatigue and poor performance! Try to eat a substantial meal at least 2-3 hours before start time. Delaying it will mean a full stomach at the start, and not only will this make you feel uncomfortable, but vital blood flow that is more useful in the muscles will be diverted to the gut. Although some competitors may swear that eating certain foods on the morning of the event improves performance, there is little supporting evidence. But, if you find that something does seem to work for you, then continue to use it. The psychology is just as important as the physical benefit.

Most of the energy for the race will come from the food eaten in the days before the event rather than the pre-event meal. In endurance races, however, some energy may be drawn from the morning meal, so try to make it high in carbohydrate content. Several enjoyable foods can provide the necessary carbohydrates. These include breakfast cereals, muffins, crumpets, toast, potato cakes, and waffles. If your anxiety level is running high, then eating may be the last thing on your agenda, but you must eat at least something, even if it is in fluid form – for example, a banana milkshake, custard, porridge or rice pudding.

Avoid fried or salted food (unless you are deliberately replacing salt losses in a hot environment). This usually leads to an uncomfortable sensation of thirst that may be troublesome on top of the dry mouth that usually comes from pre-competition nerves.

One word of warning! The morning of the event is not the time to experiment with new cereals or fibre foods. Do so at the risk of increased flatulence!

Bernie Shrosbree ...
Early starts in rallying make extra demands on the driver and co-driver. It is important to get the body and mind ready for the race by performing some light exercise, eating a light breakfast, taking a shower, and starting the hydration process for the day with sports drinks and water.

At the race venue

This is an important time for most as a good deal of mental preparation is done here. Again, stick with techniques that have worked for you in the past. Some competitors are remarkably quiet, while others prefer company. Some have been known to suddenly become religious at this point! The key is to get your body and mind ready to work at their optimum operating capacity.

In a very short time and during the race, your body will be physically subjected to jolts, bumps, and G-forces – some very sudden and unexpected. Although the training in the days leading up to the event will have prepared you for this, it is important that you prevent injury and improve performance by getting your body into optimum shape just before the start. Boxers provide a good example of physical preparation before competition. As they enter the boxing arena they are usually coated with sweat, having adequately prepared not too long before the fight. The blood flow to their muscles is optimal and they are ready for what will follow.

There are many techniques the motorsport competitor can use at this crucial time. Adequate warm-up and mobilisation of joints that will be in action is a recommended method. The advantages of a warm-up are several and were discussed in Chapter 2. A warm-up at this point will increase the blood flow, and therefore oxygen supply, to your muscles. They will then contract more efficiently, and the chances of injury will be reduced. Just as important, a good warm-up will help with mental focus and relaxation.

An adequate warm-up at the event venue may be achieved more quickly with your race suit on as this will retain the heat generated. Recommended routines include jogging on the spot or brisk walking. Lengthy routines may not be possible at race venues but it's advisable to do as much as you can, as the advantages of doing a warm-up far outweigh the disadvantages. There may be an opportunity when changing into your race suit. Swimmers usually perform stretches at this point in the privacy of the changing room, so there's no reason why you cannot do so. Some mobilisations can even be performed in the race car while waiting for the start.

Dan Clarke, World Series Champ Car driver explains his approach to warming up before a race...
It pays to warm your body up before you put it in a race car and thrash it around the track for a day. You're going to use your arms and legs without a doubt. But your core is going to get a massive workout also, not to mention your neck. Your back will also be exposed to a lot of bumps and vibrations, so a general mobilisation of the whole body will help.

In temperate climates, a total of about 15 minutes warm-up is probably sufficient before most motorsport events. If you have built up a light sweat then you have done well. Do make sure that your routine is not performed too early before the race, otherwise you will cool down. As a rule, try not to warm up longer than 30 minutes before the start.

It is important to mobilise the joints likely to be used in the event to their full range, as recommended earlier in the book. In motorsport it is the body core, arms, and neck which will take the brunt of the tremendous forces, and if the affected muscles and joints are not first moved throughout their full range prior to the race in a controlled and smooth fashion, it is highly likely that damage will occur when a jolt during the race forces them to their extreme, especially if the body is not warmed up. Remember, stretch slowly and gently but never till it causes pain.

Mental preparation

Mental preparation comes with practice. If you have been practising regularly, the mental techniques described in Chapter 7 will come easier to you at this particularly anxious time. An especially useful method is imagery or

BELOW: Dan Clarke mobilising before the start of the 2006 Long Beach event. *(Carol Loewen 2006)*

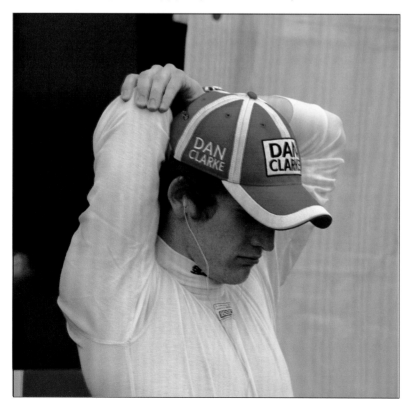

visualisation. Downhill skiers are good examples of athletes who use imagery. Just before they begin their run down the mountain, as they wait for the start buzzer, competitors can be seen with head down and eyes closed visualising their descent right up to the finish line.

Centring is also a useful technique while at the start line, especially to relieve high anxiety levels. Although a harder method to master, with practice it can dramatically reduce anxiety with only a single breath.

Louise Aitken-Walker MBE...
I just didn't go near people. I kept away from people because they can talk you into things. People can throw you off the line.

Hydration

If you get to the race venue well beforehand, start your fluid intake so you drink about 500ml (1/2 litre) around two hours before the start. This will allow any extra water to be lost as urine before the race. Then, just before the race, take in 125-250ml (1-2 small cupfuls). These are recommendations made by the American College of Sports Medicine. Try to drink as much as you comfortably can. Medical research has shown that large volumes of fluid in the stomach lead to faster emptying into the gut, which then leads to faster fluid replacement.

During the race

Even once the event has started there are ways, apart from your driving skills, to make sure you retain the edge on the competition.

It is vital that you keep well hydrated during the race. Not only does the muscular effort of driving increase body temperature, the fireproof overalls, helmets, closed cockpits, and heat radiation from the engine all make the situation worse than in most other sports. Research on Formula 1 drivers has shown sweat loss of up to 1 litre per hour while driving. In the Le Mans endurance race, drivers have been recommended to drink as much as 1.3 litres for every hour they drive.

A good way of monitoring fluid replacement is by the colour of your urine (see urine chart at the beginning of this chapter). This method is as good as laboratory methods for assessing hydration status. Aim for a pale straw-coloured urine in copious quantities. Scanty volumes of dark urine suggest dehydration. Another method is by regular weighing while racing. Aim for a replacement of 3/4 litre for every 1/2kg loss and you should be able to keep up with losses. Obviously, more fluid will be needed in hotter

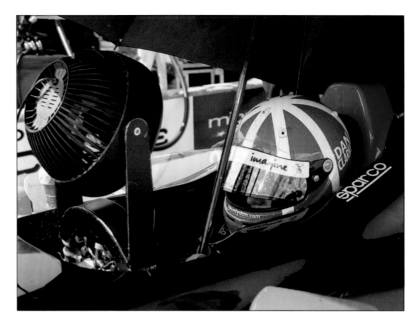

climates or if salty food is being eaten during the race. Remember that, although thirst may drive the competitor to drink, it is not the best guide to replacing fluid loss.

Drinking during racing serves two main purposes – to prevent dehydration and to provide energy. The composition of the drink will depend on which of the two you are aiming for. If you are racing for more than an hour, then use fluids with a carbohydrate content to provide energy. These have been shown to enhance performance. Commercially available sports drinks such as Red Bull, Gatorade, Isostar, and Lucozade are examples of those that provide energy. Most sports drinks contain around 7% carbohydrate, so drinking 1 litre will provide around 200-300 calories. Be aware that many 'stimulation' energy drinks, such as Red Bull, contain high levels of caffeine which make them far less effective for rehydration.

Whilst water is the obvious choice if you want to simply hydrate yourself, medical research has shown that hypotonic drinks will do the job faster. Hypotonic drinks have a lower electrolyte (salt) concentration than the body and are therefore absorbed through the gut more quickly. Most commercial sports drinks are isotonic and have the same electrolyte concentration as the body. These are absorbed as fast as, or faster than, plain water. So, if rapid replacement of fluids to counter dehydration is a priority, then go for hypotonic or even isotonic drinks rather than plain water. They will also probably be more palatable. Isotonic sports drinks are less dilute than hypotonic drinks because they contain carbohydrate for energy. They are, therefore, a

ABOVE: Dan Clarke at a World Series Champ Car race meet. He is visualising on how to approach the first corner to gain advantage. At this point the competitor's attention is totally focused on the task in hand. *(Michael Levitt, LAT USA Photography 2007)*

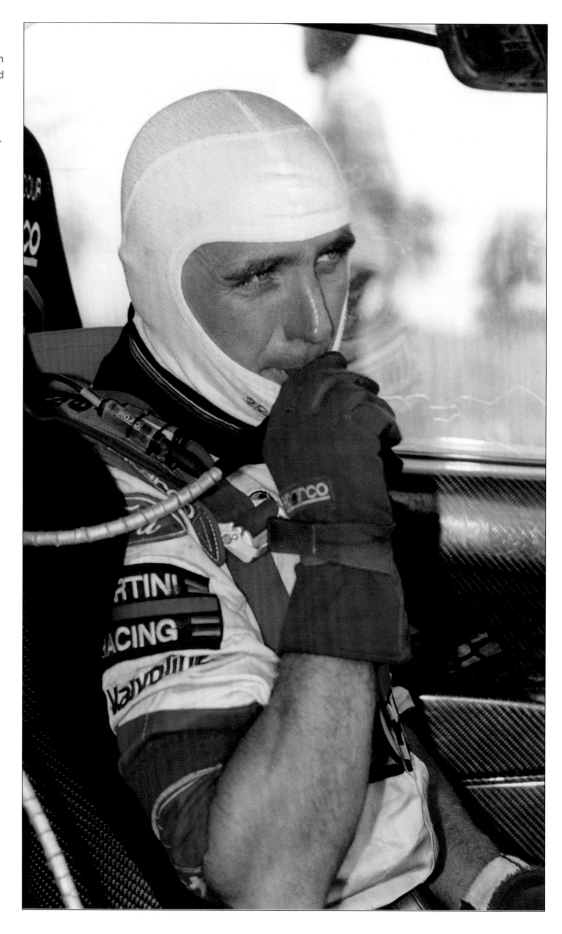

RIGHT: François Delecour, former Ford WRC driver, drinks from a flexible hose attached to a commercially available drink bladder strapped to the back of his competition seat. The spring-loaded valve, or bite-valve, easily allows regular sipping of fluids during the event. A water bottle may also be attached to the roll cage within easy access of the driver. *(Anwar Sidi, Sidi's)*

compromise between energy provision and fluid replacement.

Each competitor will have his or her own drinking preferences during competition. You are the best judge of your own drinking pattern and style. I do suggest that you try all commercially available drinks and settle with one that you like, but the day of the event is not the time to experiment. Here are some useful tips:

- Hydration status is directly related to performance, so do not ignore fluid replacement.
- Start off well hydrated. Ignore this at your peril! Once hydrated at the start you only need to top-up regularly as you lose fluids.
- Aim to maintain pale-coloured urine in reasonable quantities.
- Aim to replace every 0.5kg weight loss during competition with at least ¾ litre of fluid, i.e. always slightly higher than what you have lost.
- Remember, thirst is not the best indicator of your hydration status.
- If the race is longer than an hour, try to take in carbohydrate drinks to provide energy.
- If dehydration is a problem, choose isotonic or hypotonic drinks rather than plain water.
- Most commercial sports drinks are isotonic and are formulated to provide a balance between fluid replacement and energy provision.
- Fruit juices and fizzy drinks can initially dehydrate the body because of their high electrolyte (salt) content. They are, therefore, not ideal for rapid fluid replacement.
- If space and race format allows it, use a sports drink bladder with a flexible hose in your vehicle. Sports bottles are easy to use and have been shown to encourage drinking.
- Use cool water to make the drinks more palatable and help lower body temperature.
- Settle beforehand with a drink that you like. If none appeals to you, then make your own sports drink as shown below.
- Be aware of the dangers of hyponatraemia and over drinking too much plain water.

The table gives recommendations for the type and routine of drinking during a race.

Outside temperature is also important when it comes to the type of drink consumed. In hot climates the competitor will sweat more, and fluid replacement will be a priority over energy replacement. Hypotonic drinks will, therefore, have to be used. In the cold, isotonic drinks are more important.

Type of Race	Suggested Drinking Routine & Drink
Regular heats lasting less than 30 minutes, e.g. karting events.	Hydrate fully before race. Replace losses with water or hypotonic fluid between heats. Weigh between races if possible and assess urine colour as day progresses.
Regular races lasting longer than 30 minutes.	Hydrate fully before race. Replace losses with hypotonic drinks. Weigh between races if possible and assess urine colour as day progresses.
Races longer than an hour with regular stops, e.g. stage rallies with road sections between stages.	Hydrate fully before race. Replace losses with hypotonic fluids stored in vehicle and replace energy with isotonic carbohydrate-based drinks at service breaks. Weighing and assessment of urine colour important.
Races lasting several hours with few breaks, e.g. endurance races, long-stage rallies.	Hydrate fully before race. Replace fluid and energy losses with hypotonic fluids and isotonic carbohydrate-based drinks stored in vehicle and at pit stops. Weighing and assessment of urine colour important at beginning and end of race to replenish total losses. If not possible, aim for 1300-1500ml for every hour in the car as an approximate guide.

ABOVE: Recommended drinking patterns and content for various motorsport races.

Making your own hypotonic and isotonic drinks

Sweating is the way that the body maintains its core temperature at 37°C. However, this results in the loss of electrolytes (minerals such as calcium, chloride, magnesium, and potassium), which, if unchecked, will lead to dehydration.

Electrolytes serve 3 general functions in the body:

- Many are essential minerals
- They control osmosis of water between body compartments
- They help maintain the acid/alkaline balance needed for normal cellular activities.

There are two main factors that affect how quickly a drink gets into the body. The first is the speed at which it is emptied from the stomach, and the second is the rate at which it is absorbed through the walls of the small intestine. The higher the carbohydrate levels in the drink, the slower the rate the stomach will empty. Isotonic drinks with a carbohydrate level of between 6-8% are emptied from the stomach at a rate similar to water. Electrolytes, especially potassium and sodium, in

Commercially available isotonic and hypotonic sports drinks can be expensive. You can easily make your own, and often they are more palatable. Try the following suggestions for home-made hypotonic and isotonic sports drinks.

Isotonic drink –
ideally for energy replacement
- 200ml cordial (be sure not to use one with sweeteners) or 1 litre pure fruit juice (not juice drink)
- 1 litre water
- 1 gram (pinch) Himalayan crystal salt (Himalayan salt contains all 84 natural minerals and will not upset the balance as table salt may do)

Mix all ingredients together and keep chilled.

Hypotonic drink –
ideally for rapid fluid replacement
- 100ml cordial or 250ml pure fruit juice
- 1 litre water
- 1 gram (pinch) Himalayan crystal salt

Mix all ingredients together and keep chilled.

a drink will reduce the urine output. This enables the fluid to empty from the stomach quickly and promotes absorption in the intestines.

The best natural rehydrator is coconut water. It has a very refreshing taste and is highly thirst-quenching. In an average 330ml serving it contains zero fat, 35mg sodium, 660mg potassium, 15g carbohydrates, and 35mg magnesium. In a trial conducted by scientists in Aberdeen, it was determined that a 2% carbohydrate-electrolyte drink was more effective at combating exercise fatigue in a hot climate than a 15% mixture. (*Journal of Sports Scientist* Vol. 18, No. 5, pp339-351)

The optional addition of a small amount of salt is to provide the drinks with the necessary electrolyte balance and replace losses through sweat. Pure fruit juice is typically hypertonic (more concentrated than body fluids) so it will tend to initially dehydrate you. Carbonated drinks provide about the same rate of fluid replacement as still drinks but are associated with a higher incidence of heartburn and a bloated feeling. Most drivers prefer still drinks, but if you opt for the carbonated kind, then remember that 'diet' and 'low-calorie' drinks provide little or no energy. Their rate of fluid replacement is as fast as plain water.

What about caffeine?
Caffeine was actually a banned substance by the International Olympic Committee (IOC) Medical Commission. However, in 2004 it was removed from the banned list. Nevertheless, WADA (The World Anti Doping Agency) are currently monitoring the use of caffeine along with several other legal stimulants in sport to track patterns of usage amongst athletes.

There is no doubt that caffeine has its benefits and drawbacks when it comes to motorsport. On the positive side, most competitors and researchers will agree that it boosts concentration and mental alertness and improves reaction times. It also delays fatigue. For many it also provides a psychological prop. On the down side, it can result in anxiety and irritability, which can compound the problem of pre-competition nerves. Taken at the wrong time, caffeine can cause insomnia and deprive the competitor of much needed sleep. Possibly the most significant drawback of caffeine is its effect on dehydration. Not unusually used to kick-start the body and mind on the morning of the event by competitors who have possibly had too much alcohol the night before, it tends to further dehydrate and, therefore, impair driving performance.

Although widely used by motorsport competitors during an event, for reasons outlined above, caffeine does not necessarily improve performance and you must be aware of its diuretic effects that can work against you if you do not keep up with the replacement of fluid losses.

Caffeine usage for events should be limited to levels that you are used to and comfortable with in daily life. As with any controllable factors in your preparation, trying new strategies or products before racing should be avoided, so whilst there

BELOW: Some sports drinks, like Red Bull (45kcal/100ml), designed to provide energy, have been subjected to medical testing. This graph shows some results of a study done at the University of the West of England. Researchers found that Red Bull boosted endurance significantly compared to a control drink. (*Alford, C. et al 'The Effects of Red Bull Energy Drink on Human Performance and Mood', Amino Acids 21, 2, 139-150, 2001*)

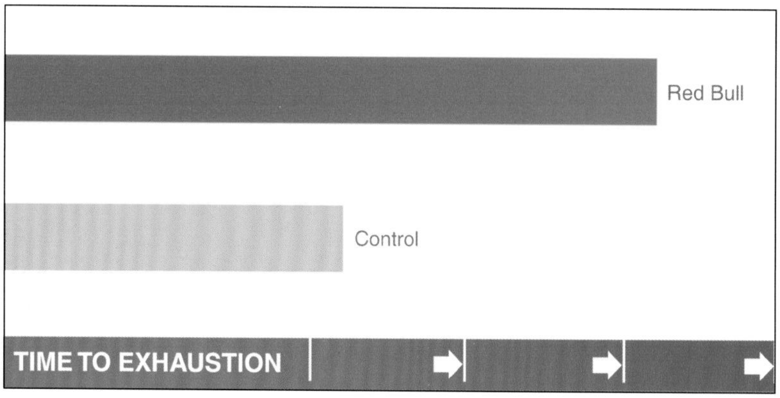

Red Bull

Control

TIME TO EXHAUSTION

is no real need to cut out or avoid caffeine when competing, overusing it, or doing so for the first time, should be avoided.

Food

To maintain performance during competition, you need the sort of solid food that will provide energy without dehydrating you excessively. The recommended and easy-to-eat foods include breakfast cereal or fruit bars, dried fruit, commercially available energy bars, bananas, and sandwiches with fillings such as jam or honey. Most solid food requires additional water to digest and process it. Make sure you take in extra water.

Food to avoid is:

- Excessively spicy food, as this can cause unpleasant reflux and discomfort.
- Excessively salty food which may result in an unpleasant sensation of thirst.
- Unfamiliar food. The day of the event is not the time to experiment with food.
- High-fibre food, especially if your body is unaccustomed to it.
- Excessively fatty food.
- Low-carbohydrate food, as this depletes the body of much needed energy.
- Difficult to digest foods, such as steaks, that may give you a bloated feeling.

Dan Clarke, Champ Car World Series driver ...

I tend to head straight for carbohydrates between sessions. Generally I'll immediately aim to replace the lost fluids after a session in the car. So an electrolyte solution will be needed, along with plenty of water. The meals I go for are generally based around fish or chicken, and I prefer a baked potato for my carbs as I find it absorbs quickly and gives me more energy than the traditional pasta/rice option other drivers go for. Greens are important too. I love broccoli, so I always make sure I can get hold of that. I prefer to have eaten just over an hour before I need to be back in the car again for qualifying or race.

Iain McPherson, Supersport biker ...

I make sure I eat about 1 1/2 hours before practice or race in order to let food digest. I try to have a balance between water and energy drinks, as drinking too much water can have an adverse affect by flushing out some of the minerals in your body, which in turn have to be replaced by supplements.

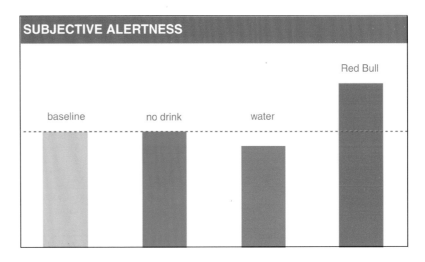

SUBJECTIVE ALERTNESS

baseline | no drink | water | Red Bull

The psychological perspective

Be at your best! Stay relaxed, be safe, keep focused on the event and let no-one and no thing distract you.

Those who have spun off during a race and have found themselves at the back of the pack will know the feelings of anger, self-directed disgust or depression that follow. Do not let such setbacks put you down and hinder your race progress. With a spin, use it as a reminder to take the same corner more skilfully next time you negotiate it. The best competitors always learn from their mistakes. If you made the error during practice you will have time to get it right in the race. If not, you can still learn as you compete. Combine the released energy from the anger you feel with some positive self-talk – 'be ready for it next time' or 'this time get the car around faster' – and you will notice the difference. You cannot be angry with yourself and at the same time give the race your best! You can, on the other hand, learn from the setback and get control of your emotions before they get control of you!

What separates the best from the rest is the ability to recover and readapt after stressful incidents. I still wonder how top Formula 1 drivers can walk away from dramatic crashes during practice and climb into the spare car within minutes to perform just as well, and sometimes better. Or how top rally drivers calmly restart their mangled cars after overturning several times, and accelerate away seemingly oblivious to the incident.

Remember this golden rule and you will do well. Potential distractions only become distractions if you let them distract you. Take them in your stride as part of the race day and they will soon be forgotten. Dwell on them, or get stressed by them, and your performance will invariably suffer. Try the

ABOVE: Red Bull contains both caffeine and taurine for their beneficial effects. Both reaction times and alertness are increased if caffeine is taken in moderation. The graph here shows that Red Bull increased alertness in 14 subjects in comparison to their baseline, with no water or water alone. *(Alford, C. et al, 'The Effects of Red Bull Energy Drink on Human Performance and Mood', Amino Acids 21, 2, 139-150, 2001)*

following tips to keep you in your stride next time you are faced with a potential distraction:

- Decide on a game plan before the race and refer to the 'bigger picture' of success every time you feel distracted.
- Remember that on race day the crowds will be bigger, competitors (including you) will be more on edge. By retaining certain expectations, you make the distractions less intrusive.
- Expect the unexpected! No competitor wants to crash during a race but the nature of the sport dictates that at some point in their careers most will. So when a crash does occur it is accepted as a risk of the sport and it fails to impact on competitor performance.
- Knowledge is power! Try to get as much information about where you are racing if you have not been there before. Ask other competitors or local clubs. Find out about the venue, the anticipated crowds, accommodation, and so on, and you will not be surprised when you turn up on race day.
- Try your level best to keep positive about the distractions. Do not waste valuable time or effort on expressing anger or disappointment in them.
- Try to begin the race in a positive frame of mind. Any distractions will have less impact if you make a good start.

There is a driver who started competing at national stage rallies with a very low budget and his car was self-prepared, under-powered in its class and was made up mostly of standard parts from the salvage yard. He was always up against better cars in his class but almost always finished events. He was also, by default, usually the top in his class. He admitted that his consistency was down to a mental game plan that he always stuck to. He would decide beforehand to run his own race and compete against no one but the clock. He was always fully aware but not flustered by the fact that others were in better cars. He knew that by trying to finish well in their class, other drivers would make mistakes. He capitalised on their errors and slowly improved his skills. Soon he was the one the crowd cheered, and in two seasons he had secured sponsorship to move on to a better car. He is a great example of someone who used positive thinking and adhered to a mental game plan to keep him physically in control.

Should a distraction affect you, then it is important your mind recovers fast. Many psychologists and team coaches purposely create distractions, such as bad calls or large noisy crowds, during training sessions to simulate what may happen during competition. Creating such distractions during motorsport can be dangerous, given the nature of the sport, so more often than not the competitor meets them for the first time on the day of the event. To learn to refocus, set some time aside beforehand to create such distractions in your mind and plan a response strategy. Settle on a plan that revolves around keeping positive, in control, and calm. Use a physical or verbal cue to get you started. Even a 'come on, let's get on with the race' may be the trigger you need, either from yourself or your co-driver, to refocus.

Dan Clarke, Champ Car World Series driver...

I find I am much more relaxed for a race if I've slept an hour before. A lot of drivers can often be found sleeping or dozing in the cockpit whilst on the grid before a race. When you've got a two-hour hard race ahead of you, there doesn't seem much point jumping around and chatting to lots of different people. I prefer to conserve energy.

If anyone knows about keeping calm during accidents and recovering from them, then its Louise Aitken-Walker. Still talked about is her famous accident at the Rally of Portugal in 1990, referred to earlier in the book, when her car slid off the road and rolled down a 150-foot cliff into a deep river. The car came to a stop upside down and fully submerged in 20 feet of water. In her own words:

We were on slick tyres and the heavens opened. I can remember we were doing well. We were coming down this bit of road, came round the corner and the car just slid. I tried to turn the steering wheel but just swished off the edge. I knew there was going to be a big accident and just thought we have to get this over with. And, of course, we rolled and rolled and rolled down the mountain. The glass was flying around and suddenly we were submerged in water. We went right to the bottom and I thought, 'I can handle this!' It was pitch black and I was hanging upside down. I was totally calm, totally calm. I undid the seatbelt and slowly came out. I tried the windscreen first but got out of the door thinking, 'I am going to live!'

This is how she regained her composure after less dramatic crashes.

The first time I crashed I couldn't believe what had happened and I was too scared to carry on. I later thought, 'Don't be stupid, you have to get over this and mentally train yourself.' I was OK and not hurt, so I needed to get going. The better you get at motorsport and the more results you get, the more hungry you get. Accidents begin to have less effect on you as long as no-one is injured. As you roll over, you start to think that the clock is ticking on. You're racing against time and that's what keeps you going.

She also offers useful advice on relaxing in the few minutes before an event.

My routine would start three minutes before the countdown at the stage start. I would get the helmet and gloves on and rest my hands in my lap. I then made tight fists, as tight as I could get them, and then relaxed. Every time I relaxed I could feel the tension leaving my body. By the time of the countdown I was ready for the stage.

After the race

This is without doubt a very important time for competitors. Even though it may be difficult, try to stick with a few basic physical and mental rules.

Make sure that you are well rehydrated. This is absolutely crucial, especially if you plan to drink any alcohol. Drink plenty of fluids, but avoid sweetened drinks in the first instance, as they tend to initially dehydrate you and over-stimulate your thirst centre. If you have been endurance racing and have lost a significant amount of sweat, consider adding a small amount of salt (¼ teaspoon to every litre of fluid) to replenish any sodium salts that you will have lost.

Try to avoid alcohol if you are injured during the race. The short-term treatment of acute injuries is to reduce the inflammatory process that follows by applying rest, ice, compression, and elevation to the affected area. Alcohol acts in the opposite manner and makes injuries worse.

Make sure that you replenish the glycogen in the used muscles soon after the race. A rapid way of doing this is to drink a carbohydrate-rich drink that would also provide the water if dehydrated. Try also to eat a carbohydrate-rich meal if you can. The ingestion of food also serves to absorb any alcohol that you drink after the race. Suitable foods include pasta, baked potatoes, rice, and noodles.

Bear in mind that competitors may be tested for drugs and alcohol up to 30 minutes after a race, and that the prescribed limit is zero.

BELOW: Fitness in action. Guiding the driver after downpours made certain sections impassable. *(Anwar Sidi Images)*

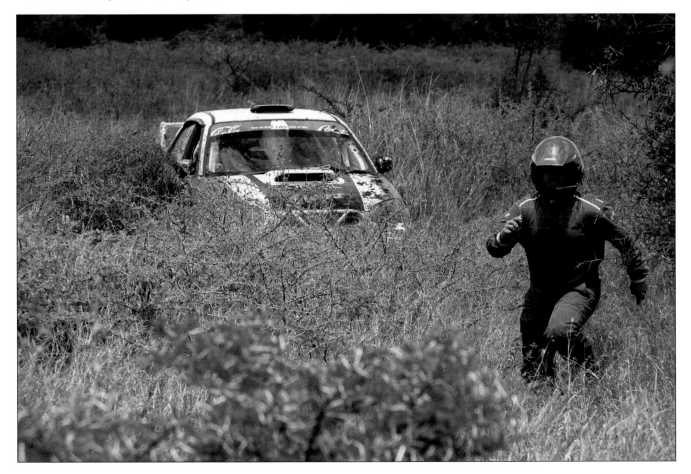

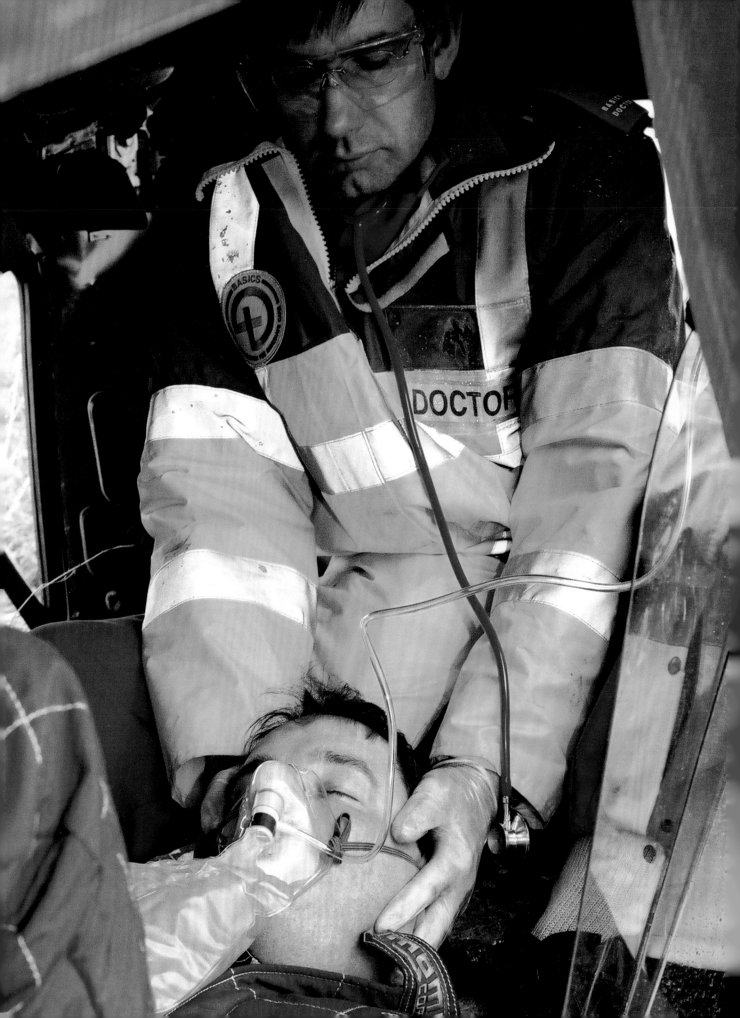

12

Emergency care in motorsport

It is surprising how little competitors know of what to do in the event of an emergency and about what rescue procedures will be put into operation should they become an accident victim.

This chapter provides the reader with the fundamentals of basic life support (BLS) and other immediate care principles, which should be observed whilst waiting for the medical crew to arrive, and it explains what may happen to a competitor during a rescue attempt. Vital time may be lost through an accident victim's ignorance of rescue procedures and the equipment used. Already in shock, they may be so frightened by what is happening to them that the rescue team's efforts are hindered.

Formal training in First Aid or, as a minimum, BLS, is recommended. In Britain, courses are available through such organisations as the Red Cross and St John Ambulance, as well as a number of commercial organisations.

At its most basic level, life requires a patient to be breathing oxygen, and pumping that oxygen around their body to vital organs such as the brain, heart, and lungs. The aim of BLS is to support the casualty's airway, breathing, and circulation (conveniently labelled A, B and C in that order of priority) using no aids. BLS aims to preserve blood flow to the brain and other vital organs, while waiting for definitive medical care.

Unless you are privileged to be driving Formula 1 or Indy car circuits it may take rescue and medical crews a few minutes to reach the scene of the accident. In British rallying, for example, the requirement is for rescue and medical services to be placed at the start of a special

stage, or at a suitable mid-point if it is more than nine miles long. In some long-stage World Championship events, such as the Safari Rally, where stage distances of up to 140km (90 miles) are not uncommon, bad crashes can occur in remote places and it can be some time before an accident is discovered. In such cases the survival of the injured depends on those who first come upon the scene and on their ability to apply BLS and other important first-aid principles.

Accident assessment

Carefully inspect the accident scene and make sure that it is safe to approach. Do not needlessly expose yourself to dangers, and remember many are not immediately obvious. In circuit racing this may be other race traffic that not uncommonly head into a crashed car still on the track. In rallies there may be another vehicle seconds behind. There may be spilled fuel and the car may still be running. Every attempt should be made to turn off the engine and the electrical isolator switch on the outside of the vehicle before approaching the casualty. There may be a fire that needs to be put out before any rescue attempt can be made. Also make sure that you are wearing sufficient clothing to protect you from fuel or blood spills.

Once you consider the scene safe to approach, you can inspect the casualty. If possible, approach the casualty from the front of the vehicle to get their attention. This will reduce the risk of them turning their head to see you, which may exacerbate any neck injuries they may have.

OPPOSITE: On long-stage rallies it may take some time for the medical professionals to arrive. *(Roger Bell)*

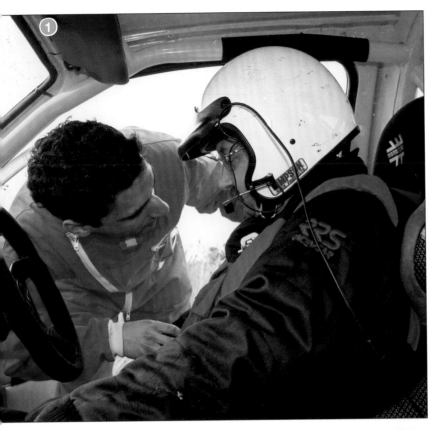

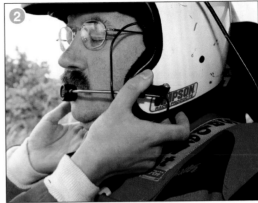

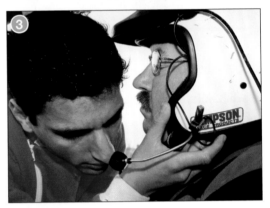

Initial assessment of someone injured.
1) Approach from the front if possible.
2) Lift jaw if casualty is unconscious or if airway sounds compromised.
3) Check for breathing by looking, listening, and feeling in one simple manoeuvre.
4) Administer rescue breathing. *(Roger Bell)*

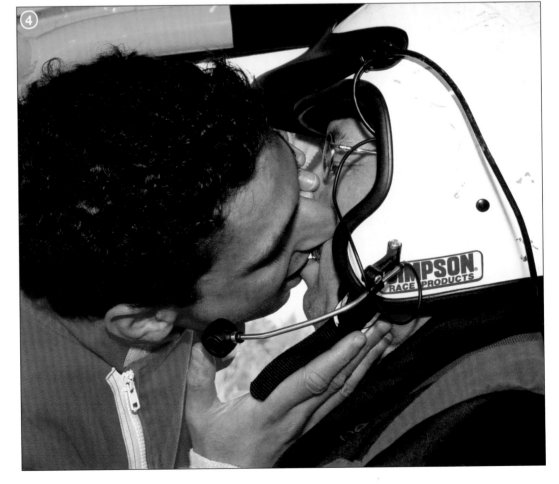

It is then appropriate to speak to the driver, asking 'Are you okay?' If the answer is sensible and in a normal voice then you can reasonably assume at that stage, that:

- the airway is open and clear,
- breathing is sufficient to reply, and …
- circulation of blood to the brain is enough for a sensible answer to be given.

Remember that these assumptions only indicate the casualty's present condition. There can be a sudden deterioration at any time during the rescue attempt, so make sure you reassess them regularly until help arrives. In the meantime, leave them in the position you find them provided they are not in further danger.

If the casualty is unconscious or if there are gurgling, wheezing, snoring or abnormal noises coming from their airway, the airway must be opened and cleared as explained below.

If you are a marshal or a competitor in an area where there are other officials about, you can ask one of them to summon rescue services once you have made the above brief assessment. This should be done through a nearby radio operator if at all possible. Accurate concise information about the type of accident, number of casualties involved, who is injured (whether competitors and/or spectators), and precise details on location should be provided if possible.

If the location is more remote (for example in a rally event) and you are alone, then if needed you should provide BLS for as long as possible and flag down a passing competitor's car and get them to pass on the above information. They should stop anyway if they see an SOS board (see later). Do not worry about affecting their race time as account will be taken of this later if they have stopped for this reason. If you know that there will be no further race cars following, then perform the life saving manoeuvres for about a minute before going for help. If BLS is required, this measure is only ever a 'stop-gap' to keep the brain and heart oxygenated prior to definitive medical care, so this care must be summoned in some way.

At a motorsport event, mobile phones should only be used as a last resort as confusion can arise if messages come through the 999 system rather than the established safety channels.

(A) Airway

This takes priority when dealing with anyone who is injured. If the casualty is unconscious, the airway will probably be compromised as the tongue falls back and obstructs the opening to the windpipe. In an upright crashed car the unconscious competitor may be slumped forward shutting off the airway. Check and remove any obvious obstructions from their mouth, such as chewing gum, loose dentures, vomit or broken teeth. CAREFULLY lifting the jaw forwards (also known as jaw thrust) usually opens the airway by elevating the tongue off the back of the airway. It is important that you do this carefully, as excessive force can cause damage to the spinal cord in the neck, especially if there is a neck fracture. AVOID LIFTING THE CHIN OR TILTING THE HEAD. Once the jaw is lifted, look for signs and listen for sounds of improved breathing as the airway is opened.

Although these manoeuvres are standard practice when resuscitating other casualties, they have severe limitations in the case of an injured unconscious competitor. The limitations are discussed in the following section.

If the casualty is wearing a full-face helmet, open the visor to improve air flow. If the chin strap is digging deeply into the neck, it may be shutting off the airway. Carefully loosen the strap, but avoid taking the helmet off.

What about suspected neck injuries?

Following any accident, an unconscious patient, or a patient who has suffered a high-speed impact with substantial vehicle damage, especially to front and rear end, MUST be assumed to have a spinal injury to the neck. This injury can be fatal. The great Ferrari driver Gilles Villeneuve, father of Jacques Villeneuve, died of such an injury after a crash during practice at Zolder in Belgium in 1982.

While trained race rescuers know what actions to perform with a suspected neck injury, it is important that bystanders or fellow competitors do not inadvertently cause any further damage. Here's a checklist of what to do, and what not to do, before the medical and rescue crew arrive:

- If at all possible, try to approach the casualty from the front. This means the casualty does not have to move their head to reply to you. Any head movement is risking further spinal damage.
- Avoid chin lift or head tilt when opening the airway. These moves can damage the spinal cord if there is an unstable neck fracture already present. CAREFULLY use jaw thrust as the primary manoeuvre. LIMITED head tilt must only be used in life-threatening situations, for example if the jaw thrust alone is insufficient to

open the airway. In this situation the patient will certainly die of airway obstruction if the head is not moved. If it is necessary to move the head, the degree of movement should be all that is required to open the airway, and no more.

■ Avoid moving the casualty excessively unless the situation warrants immediate removal – from a burning car, for example.

■ Do not try to remove the helmet, except if it is necessary to do so, in order to gain access to the patient's airway. This is especially important if there is substantial damage to the helmet, or if there is blood seeping from the head area. Helmet removal requires trained personnel, usually including a doctor or paramedic.

■ Always speak to the casualty explaining what you are doing even if they are unconscious. It calms and reassures them.

If the car is on fire and the flames are beginning to get out of control, you will have to balance the risks. Under such circumstances any reasonable action to immediately move the casualty out of danger is considered appropriate. When doing this, try to keep the casualty's head supported at all times. Avoid tilting it backwards if at all possible.

(B) Breathing

Once the airway is cleared, maintain the position without excessive movement of the head until help arrives. Also check that the casualty is breathing normally, i.e. there is more than just the occasional gasp.

To check for breathing follow this routine for ten seconds:

■ LOOK for the chest moving,
■ LISTEN close to the casualty's mouth for breath sounds, and …
■ FEEL for breath on your cheek.

All three actions can be performed in one simple manoeuvre.

If the casualty is breathing spontaneously, maintain the airway until help arrives and move on to checking circulation. Keep checking regularly to ensure that the breathing does not deteriorate.

If the casualty is not breathing, then you must breathe for them. Make sure first that someone has already called for help. Check once again and remove any obvious obstructions from the casualty's mouth. To start ventilation deliver

two effective breaths using mouth-to-mouth ventilation. You may have up to five attempts to deliver these two breaths, before you should move on to a further assessment.

This ventilation gives the casualty around 16% oxygen from your expired breath compared to 21% that is available from normal atmospheric air. It is also known as 'rescue breathing'.

This technique is not easy, and professional training is recommended to familiarise the rescuer with the methods required to perform it. To perform it effectively the following method is suggested:

■ Keep the casualty's airway open by using jaw thrust but avoiding chin lift and head tilt.

■ Pinch the soft part of the nose with the index finger and thumb of one hand. This would be your right hand if rescuing a casualty from the left-hand seat of a crashed vehicle.

■ Open the casualty's mouth slightly, maintaining jaw thrust.

■ Having taken a deep breath, seal your lips around the casualty's mouth.

■ Exhale steadily for about two seconds and look for the chest rising. Although difficult to judge, you are aiming to deliver around ¾ to 1 litre of breath.

■ Allow the casualty to empty their lungs, maintaining the airway at all times. This should take about three seconds.

■ Take a deep breath before each ventilation to ensure you deliver the best possible oxygen concentration.

Important notes

■ If there is much resistance, then assume that the airway must still be compromised. Check in the mouth for any vomit, blood or obvious obstructions. If any are present take care in removing them, as the situation can be worsened by inadvertently forcing them further down the airway. Make sure you have an effective seal when breathing into the casualty's mouth. There should be little resistance when performing effective mouth-to-mouth ventilation.

■ Ventilating too rapidly may cause air to inflate the stomach rather than the lungs.

■ Using large volumes of breath may also cause the stomach to inflate.

■ If there is blood or vomit in the mouth, severe jaw injury, or if the rescuer's hand is not free to keep the nose pinched shut, it is acceptable to perform mouth-to-nose ventilation. In this case, seal your mouth around the casualty's nose and follow the steps outlined above. Remember to open the mouth when the casualty exhales. Mouth-to-nose ventilation may not be possible with severe nose injuries or with extensive damage to cheekbones.

■ Make at least five attempts to provide two effective breaths. Do not waste too much time on any more. Move on to the assessment of the circulation.

(C) Circulation

Assessment and management of the circulation involves two key elements. The first is to examine for the presence of an effective circulation, and to support it if necessary. The second is to control any major bleeding to conserve the casualty's own blood.

In the past, resuscitation guidelines for lay people recommended that circulation should be assessed by feeling for a major pulse, such as the carotid pulse in the neck or femoral pulse in the groin for at least 10 seconds. While this remains true for professional rescuers, recent guidelines from leading organisations, such as the European Resuscitation Council, now recommend that lay and non-professional rescuers should simply 'look for signs of circulation'. This recommendation followed studies that showed that even experienced rescuers can make mistakes when feeling for a major pulse.

It is now agreed that for the non-professional or lay person, an assessment of circulation should include:

■ Giving two effective rescue breaths.
■ Looking, listening, and feeling for normal breathing, coughing or movement for no longer than 10 seconds.

If you are sure that the casualty has good signs of circulation, then continue ventilating until they start breathing normally. Remember that the casualty can deteriorate at any time, so check regularly.

If there are no signs of circulation, or you are unsure, then the casualty's heart has stopped working effectively and you must start chest compressions to get the blood circulating. For this you will need the help of someone else to hold the airway open and/or even perform rescue breathing. It may be impossible to perform the breathing and compressions in the confines of a racing cockpit, or if you are alone. In this case it may be reasonable to extricate the casualty, with due attention to the neck, and

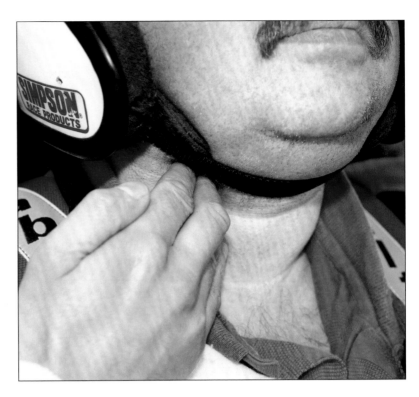

undertake life support with the casualty on their back.

Chest compressions

■ Locate where the ribs meet in the front of the chest. This is the lower part of the sternum bone, which extends to the top of the chest where it meets the neck.
■ Place the heel of one hand over the lower third of the sternum.
■ Place the heel of the first hand over the other and interlock the fingers.
■ Lean over the casualty so that your shoulders are directly over your hands with your arms fully straightened.
■ Firmly and smoothly press straight down on the breastbone so that it depresses about 4-5cm (1½-2 inches).
■ Release the pressure, keeping your hand on the breastbone so your position does not change.
■ Repeat the compressions, aiming for a rate of about 100 per minute, or just slower than two compressions a second.

Important Dos and Don'ts

Do:

■ Make sure that the chest compression time is at least 50% of each cycle (see later).
■ Check for signs of circulation if the casualty makes a sudden movement or takes a breath, as the heart may have started to work.

ABOVE: Locating the carotid pulse in a casualty. It is now recommended that only professional rescuers should use this to assess circulation. Lay persons and non-professional rescuers must look for signs of circulation as described in the text of this book. *(Roger Bell)*

Chest compressions.
1) Locating the xiphisternal notch in front of the chest where the ribs meet.
2) Placing the heel of the other hand two finger-breadths above the xiphisternal notch.
3) Interlocking the fingers of both hands to provide an effective method of chest compression.
4) Effective positioning over the casualty with arms straight and shoulders over the breastbone.
(Roger Bell)

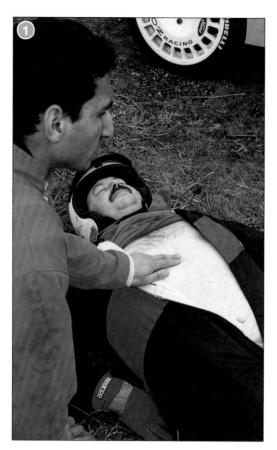

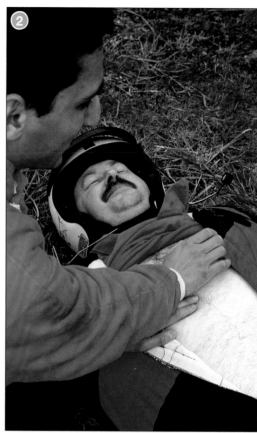

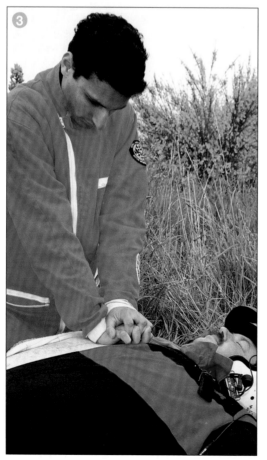

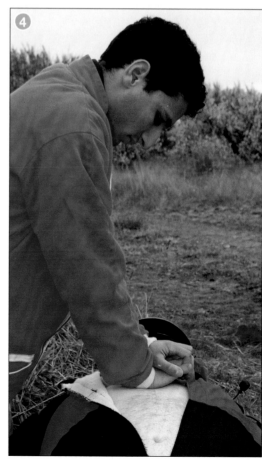

Don't:

■ Apply sudden jerky movements, and try to avoid bending your elbows.
■ Interrupt ventilation and compression unless checking for signs of circulation. Even in that case, take no more than 10 seconds.
■ Assume that feeling a pulse while doing chest compressions indicates the return of normal heart function. You are probably feeling the pressure wave from the compression.

Organising the rescuers

One-person rescue:

It is difficult to decide when to get help and how much life support to perform, if any, before seeking help. There is no one answer as it depends largely on the situation. Generally speaking in trauma, however, help should be summoned after adequate resuscitation has been in place for about a minute.

A single rescuer must aim to provide 30 chest compressions after giving the initial two expired air ventilation breaths. This cycle must then be repeated.

Two-person rescue:

This is more effective than single-rescue BLS, as the chest compressions are not interrupted for as long. Two-person rescue may follow on from single-person rescue as someone returns from getting help.

Two-person rescue must also aim to provide 30 chest compressions for every two breaths provided. The chest compressions must pause for only as long as it takes to provide two breaths.

The guidelines changed at the end of 2005, to recommend 30 compressions per two ventilations for all adult BLS scenarios, irrespective of the number of rescuers. This is following evidence indicating that more chest compressions have a greater efficiency in providing a blood supply to the brain and heart.

Performing BLS, especially chest compressions, is a very tiring procedure. Where possible, it is important to change rescuers every minute or two, to reduce fatigue, which has been shown to reduce the efficiency of chest compressions.

Control of bleeding

The casualty with major bleeding will die from blood loss, in spite of efforts to support A, B, and C. Once the body has lost a significant proportion of blood, the ability to carry oxygen is reduced, and damage to the organs will result.

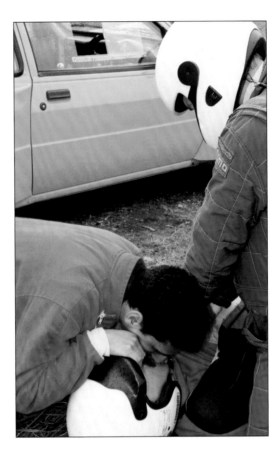

LEFT: Two-person BLS.
(Roger Bell)

Blood loss may occur from a number of injuries, and may be internal or external. Little can be done for internal bleeding in the first-aid environment, except summoning help to facilitate rapid transfer to hospital.

Attempts can be made to control external bleeding using pressure to wounds, in much the same way that we will squeeze our nostrils together to control a nosebleed, or place a sticky plaster over a cut.

A major wound with blood flowing from it represents a significant threat to life. The simplest measure to reduce bleeding is to place a dressing (ideally a sterile first-aid dressing, but failing that any absorbent material, such as a torn item of clothing) directly into or on to the wound, then to apply direct pressure firmly and continuously to the wound. If blood seeps through this dressing, a second dressing should be placed over, and direct pressure applied again.

If these efforts fail, the next step, where possible, is to apply pressure higher up the limb where the blood supply comes from. However, unless you have received training in these methods, continuous application of direct pressure is likely to be the safest and most effective measure to employ.

RIGHT: The results of
the fiery accident in the
1976 German Grand
Prix that left Niki Lauda
scarred.

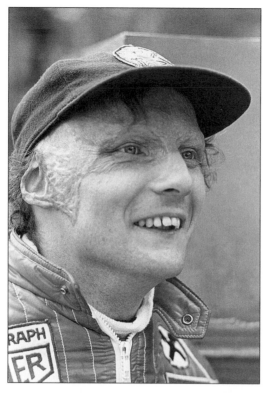

BELOW: Being trapped
in a burning car is
probably a competitor's
biggest nightmare.
(Anwar Sidi Images)

What about burns?

Any competitor's biggest nightmare must be
being trapped and unconscious in their rally or
race car when it catches fire. This happened to
Niki Lauda who suffered extensive facial burns in
his accident in the 1976 German Grand Prix at
Nürburgring. Amazingly, though, he escaped and
went on to win the World Driver's title in 1977,
and again in 1984.

FIA regulations for fire safety are justifiably very
strict for all types of events, and every competitor
should get the best fire safety equipment
affordable.

The approach to the accident vehicle on fire
depends on the vehicle and event involved.
In circuit and race meetings, such as karting,
saloon car racing, and even Formula racing,
there are strategically placed fire safety officials
and marshals as the first line of attack. In
stage rallying, however, the responsibility lies
with the competitors or even the spectators.
Most regulations insist on having a master
circuit-breaker placed within arm's reach of the
competitors, and also located externally. These

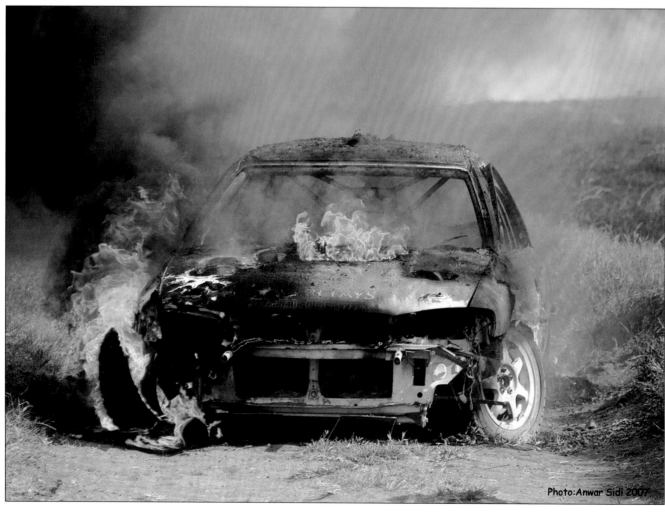

Photo:Anwar Sidi 2007

breakers, which are usually cable-operated, isolate all electrical circuits of the race car, with exception of those required to operate the fire extinguishers, thereby minimising the risk of fire. The external breaker is usually mounted on the lower part of the windscreen on the driver's side. Occasionally it may be found by the rear window. In open cars it is located on the driver's side at the lower end of the main roll-over bar or at the bottom of the windscreen. The breaker is marked by a red spark on a white-edged blue triangle. The 'ON' and 'OFF' positions should be clearly marked.

All racing vehicles carry a fire extinguisher or extinguishing system capable of being activated by the competitor in an emergency. The minimum requirements again depend upon the vehicle and event type. Generally, extinguishers may be hand-held or plumbed-in. They may also be manually or electrically activated. No vehicle should pass scrutineering before the race unless it meets the minimum requirements laid down by the ASN.

As with the circuit-breaker, the fire system may be triggered externally by marshals, spectators or competitors themselves. The trigger should be located next to, or in some cases combined with, the circuit-breaker. It is marked by the letter 'E' in red on a white circle.

Dealing with burns

As with other forms of rescue, do not attempt to rescue a casualty until a fire, or the risk of a fire, has been dealt with effectively. Remember that, although the fire itself may have been doused, the casualty may still be burning because of smouldering clothes. Burns casualties are likely also to suffer more breathing complications than others, not only because of inhaled smoke but also because of heat injury to their airways.

Beware of those with facial burns or soot around their nostrils or in their spit. These indicate that the airway has been burned, and later swelling may result in severe breathing problems.

Any casualties involved in a vehicle fire need to be seen by rescue and medical personnel, even though they may think they are uninjured at that early stage. Casualties with a wheeze or hoarse voice, or difficulty swallowing, may be suffering respiratory problems which can develop hours after the event. It is also possible for drivers suffering from smoke inhalation to suffer from carbon monoxide poisoning. Both of these scenarios are usually dealt with relatively easily and safely, if medical attention is sought immediately, but may be difficult to treat if they present late.

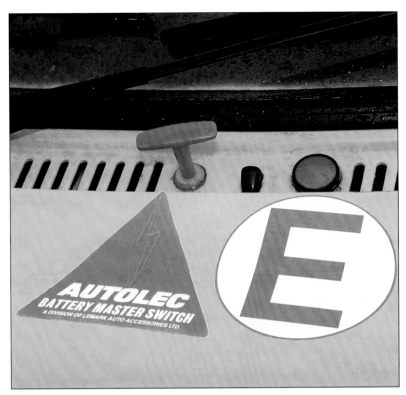

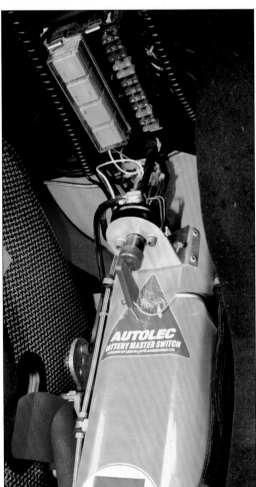

ABOVE AND LEFT:
Externally and internally mounted circuit-breaker and fire-extinguishing system trigger on a rally car.
(Roger Bell)

Important Dos and Don'ts

Do:

- Remove clothing likely to continue the burning process, such as smouldering or those saturated with hot liquids.
- Remove clothing saturated with fuel or battery acid, as chemical burns can be very painful.
- Remember that burnt areas swell rather quickly, so cut away or remove clothing likely to constrict.
- Make sure the casualty is kept warm, especially if large amounts of water have been used to treat the burns.

Don't:

- Become a casualty yourself – your safety is of paramount importance.
- Remove clothes stuck to burnt skin.
- Burst any blisters that may form.
- Apply excessive amounts of cold soaks or ice packs, as the casualty may become hypothermic, especially in casualties with massive burns.

What competitors should expect

Overall, motorsport accidents today are relatively uncommon considering the speed and popularity of the sport, and this is mainly because of the safety measures now mandatory with most forms of the sport. When accidents do occur, any emergency is normally handled promptly and effectively by well-trained rescue and medical crews.

However, it is important that drivers are aware of standard emergency procedures. When trapped and in pain, most people will exhibit a 'fight or flight' response, especially if they are in shock or drifting in and out of consciousness. But if they are familiar with rescue crew routine, even if the communicating language is not in their mother tongue, they are more likely to cooperate than hinder progress by struggling. They will learn to expect certain questions from the rescue and medical staff, and they will effectively take part in their own rescue.

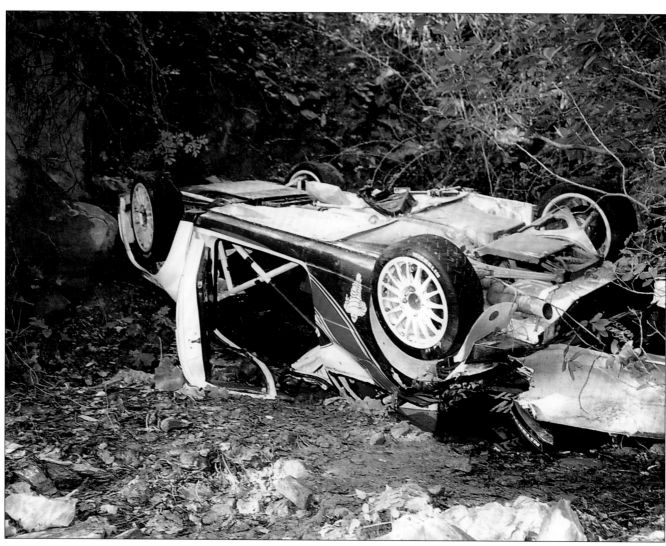

BELOW: The notorious Corsica Rally claims yet another casualty. Colin McRae's and Nicky Grist's infamous crash that led to some questions being asked about provision of rescue services at certain rally events. *(Maurice Selden, Martin Holmes Rallying)*

If trapped and conscious

Motorsport accidents occur so quickly that there is little that can be done until the car comes to a stop. Only then can an account be taken of what has happened.

A driver's initial thoughts (invariably following a few choice words) are usually those of disbelief. Then their own safety becomes a priority as they take stock of what state they (and their co-driver if present) are in. Pain will probably not be felt immediately because of the levels of adrenaline and other hormones in their system. Most then try to scramble free from their car fearing fire or being crashed into by following cars, and if they find they are trapped there is a tendency to panic, and most will struggle to free themselves from whatever is trapping them. It is at this point that the pain of any injury will be felt.

How the driver is trapped will depend on the type of crash. With head-on accidents, the footwell may buckle on to the feet, or the steering wheel and column may move towards the torso. In saloon car rollovers, the roof may have buckled, severely limiting movement within the cockpit.

When will help arrive?

The response times and the make up of the emergency units present at the event will depend upon the event type and the regulations laid down by the ASN.

As an example, in Britain at a race or speed event, Race Rescue Units with a doctor or MSA-registered paramedic aim to be at the scene of the accident within about 90 seconds of being deployed. Marshals will also have attended the scene, and will probably be with the driver within a few seconds.

At multi-use stage rallies there will be a similar Rally Rescue Unit, as well as a Recovery Unit at each stage start. Stages longer than nine miles will have a similar set-up at a suitable mid-point. These all are minimum requirements, and in many cases higher standards will be achieved. Nonetheless, this will likely result in a significantly longer response time for the emergency services on a rally sector incident, compared with a race circuit incident.

The Rescue Unit

This vehicle is a fully equipped ambulance able to carry at least one fully immobilised casualty, and probably one other 'walking wounded'. It has much of the equipment a standard county ambulance would have, with additional advanced life support equipment for use by the associated paramedic or doctor. It also carries tools for facilitating safe

extrication described later in this section. The personnel are trained and experienced in race or rally marshalling, advanced first-aid, and in the handling of all the cutting equipment.

The Recovery Unit

Traditionally, this vehicle tidied up at the end of a rally stage or race, recovering wrecks after the stage was over, and towing them out. Like many of the safety disciplines in modern motorsport, the crews have become much more professional and now have an important role in the primary response, providing additional vehicle stabilisation and dismantling skills. Also, extra pairs of experienced hands are always useful at an incident.

While accidents are rapidly detected at speed and circuit events, during multi-use stage rallies it may take several minutes before the rescue and medical teams are notified and mobilised. If not already reported over the radio or mobile phone by the competitors themselves, the following race cars will usually report the accident to race officials

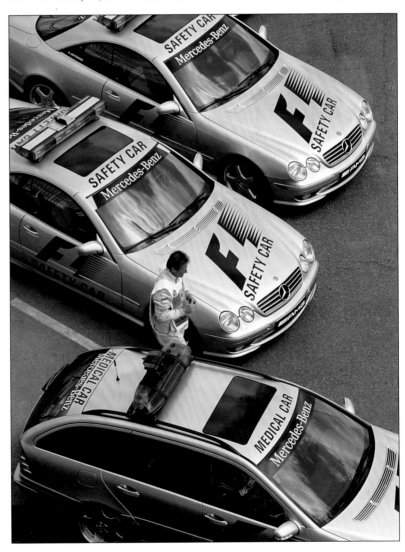

BELOW: The Race Rescue Unit on standby at a Formula 1 race meeting. *(Mike Gibbon, MVG Photographic)*

at the stage finish. In the UK, all competitors are required to carry an A4 size white board with a red coloured SOS on one side and a green OK on the other. The SOS should be displayed to following competitors if medical assistance is required and the OK if the crew is safe.

It may happen to you

If you are unfortunate enough to crash, and find yourself trapped, it is important that you try to keep calm. Take stock of what injuries, if any, you have sustained and think of how you can aid your own rescue.

Try to apply to yourself, if possible, the same principles of Airway, Breathing, and Circulation mentioned earlier in this section. How is your breathing (or that of your co-driver)? Take a deep and gentle breath in. Is that painful? If so it could indicate damage to your ribs and chest wall. Try to avoid taking your helmet off and moving your head excessively in case you have an undiagnosed neck fracture. Keep your head in a neutral position, and especially avoid tilting your head back or forwards. A neck fracture may sound impossible, but I have dealt with a fully conscious casualty after a road traffic accident who was discovered to have an unstable neck fracture several hours after his transfer to hospital. In fact, he had already been through the local hospital before being transferred by helicopter to our surgical team. During that time no attention had been paid to his neck. He was very fortunate to have no resulting damage. This goes to show that such injuries may be difficult to diagnose, and should always be assumed to be present until they can be excluded by appropriately trained personnel.

Do you have any tingling sensations or weakness in your limbs? Any localised pain will probably give you a fair idea of what you have injured. Very gently try to move your legs and feet, as they are the most likely to be trapped. If you have any severe pain or can feel abnormal grating sensations, then stop as this could indicate fractures. Try also not to twist your spine too much as you wait for help, especially if doing so causes numbness and tingling in your limbs. Qualified rescue crews are trained to suspect a spinal injury in all such accidents and will extricate you from the vehicle using special equipment designed to keep your spine protected at all times.

Also, try to take stock of how safe the vehicle is for those trying to rescue you. An early priority of a rescue crew chief who controls a rescue attempt is to ensure stability of the vehicle. You can aid this process by telling him whether the car is precariously balanced or safe to approach. Also let him know if there has been a fuel spill or if you managed to isolate the race car electrics after the accident.

It is important that the attending medical staff also know whether you have suffered any burns, or if you were exposed to any smoke. As eluded to earlier, burns and suspected smoke inhalation injuries require special care and management that is best started early.

There will be questions that the doctor or paramedic may also ask you. These will be about whether you have any allergies, your tetanus status, the last time you had anything to eat or drink, and any significant medical history they should be aware of.

Almost certainly the first question you will be asked will be 'Are you OK?' As a member of a race rescue crew it is reassuring to be told, 'I'm OK! I don't think I was knocked out. I'm sore when I breathe in deeply on the right side of my chest, though. I can't move my right leg – I think it is trapped!', or something along those lines. Not only does that indicate that the casualty has a patent airway, adequate breathing, and reasonable blood circulation to the brain, they have taken account of what has happened to them and what needs attention. On the other hand, an aggressive and uncooperative casualty may be an indication of advanced blood loss or some other life-threatening medical condition, that necessitates immediate removal and attention, probably not in the smooth and painless manner that would have otherwise been the case.

Who will get to you first?

This depends largely on the event type and regulations local to you. In the UK, for example, the emergency unit may consist of the Medical and Race Rescue Unit in the same vehicle. Many

BELOW: The red SOS card displayed prominently on the car for the attention of passing vehicles. The OK sign is green. (Roger Bell)

rally and hill climb events have this set up. In some circuit events, such as Formula 1 races, there may be a Fast Doctor Car that acts as a first response unit and provides immediate casualty care while the Rescue Unit is on its way. Recently First Intervention Vehicles (FIVs) have been introduced to international rallying and also to some circuit events. Like Fast Doctor Cars they provide basic casualty care until the Race Rescue Unit arrives. Occasionally a Snatch Vehicle may be employed to move the stranded accident vehicle from danger before any attention can be paid to the casualty.

The Race Rescue Unit

The Race Rescue Unit normally consists of a crew chief, two tool operators and a spare man who may also double up as an assistant to the doctor. Their services are normally voluntary. The unit is led by the crew chief, whose role is essentially to control and co-ordinate the rescue attempt. He will be the one directing the rescue crew and delegating tasks. If there is no doctor or paramedic present he will allocate a member of the team to fulfil that role while he makes an initial assessment of the scene, its safety, and vehicle damage. He will then report to the doctor the condition of the casualty, nature of entrapment, and preferred method and speed of extrication.

If the entrapment is complex, the crew chief's priority is to ensure scene safety, and then to create enough space for the medical crew to work in and stabilise the casualty. Once the extrication plan is decided on, the chief then stabilises the vehicle, if required, by means of ropes, props or belts. Generally, assuming the crew is sufficient and competent, the chief will have to do little 'hands-on' work, lending only the occasional hand. His role is essentially supportive and supervisory.

The equipment

The aim of using equipment is to create enough space in a safe manner so that the trapped and injured casualty can be removed without further harm and damage.

Race Rescue Units carry a tremendous amount of equipment designed to extricate even the most awkwardly trapped casualty. The equipment can be broadly classified as either powered or hand tools. Once the extrication plan is decided, one member of the team will be assigned to assemble the heavier power tools while the others will probably begin work using hand tools such as hacksaws and Stanley knives. Before any work is started, however, the casualty will be protected from flying debris either by plastic transparent shields or blankets.

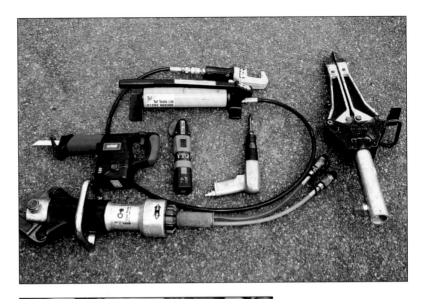

ABOVE: Some of the power-tools likely to be encountered during a rescue attempt – electric saw, pneumatic air chisel, combination cutters and spreaders, and a helmet saw. *(Roger Bell)*

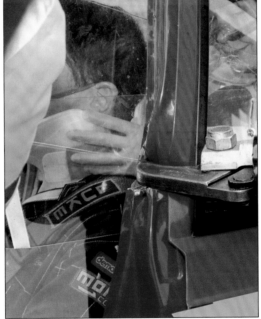

LEFT: The combination hydraulically-operated cutter and spreader seen cutting through a door pillar and roll cage of a competition car with apparent ease. *(Roger Bell)*

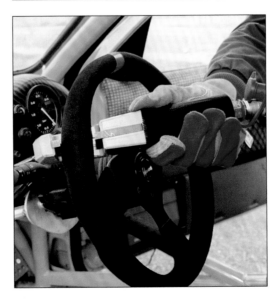

LEFT: Hydraulically-operated pedal cutters for cutting through a steering wheel. *(Roger Bell)*

Electric generators, bottled air or hydraulics may power the tools. In either case they are extremely noisy, especially when working in a confined space as they are likely to be. The types of powered tools found in Race Rescue Units commonly include air or electric saws, helmet saws, air chisels (Zip guns), spreaders, and cutters.

The saws are versatile and can be used for cutting through pillars of the accident vehicle. They generate a fair amount of vibration and noise, and if close to the casualty may cause nausea and vomiting. Air chisels are normally used for cutting through door panels, while combination cutters and spreaders, either hand or power operated, are useful for bursting open hinges or cutting through most materials. They are extremely powerful tools that are treated with utmost respect by the rescue crew. Although the jaws move slowly, they exert extremely high pressures that can be difficult to control. It is, therefore, essential that you keep well clear of their working ends.

Other hydraulic tools include pedal cutters, designed to free trapped feet from distorted foot wells and cut through steering wheels, and rams that can lift collapsed engine bulkheads that commonly result from front-end impacts. As the pedal cutter will be used in close proximity to the trapped casualty it is essential that the casualty cooperates fully to prevent injury. While the hydraulic tools are being operated, depending on the type of tool being used, you may hear various commands such as 'pump' and 'release' being shouted to the pump operator by the rescuer positioning the working ends of the tool.

In some rare cases it will be necessary to cut the helmet from a conscious casualty using a helmet saw. The cutting blade of a helmet saw is usually circular. It oscillates at a high frequency and only cuts when applied to a solid object. It will therefore not cut into human skin or tissue unless the blade is pressed on skin over a bone, e.g. the jaw. If such a tool is being used on you, please try to cooperate fully with the rescuer. Application of the saw blade to the helmet is very noisy and results in vibrations that may disorientate you. The rescue crew will try to make this as brief as possible for you, and this method will only be used if it is not possible to remove your helmet using the normal method, either owing to damage to the helmet, or if it is necessary to protect you from further injury.

Basic extrication strategies

The strategies discussed below are largely relevant to motorsport vehicles that resemble conventional road going vehicles. The principles of extrication are, however, the same for all other forms of racing vehicles.

To gain access to the casualty and ensure their safe removal, the accident vehicle can be entered either through the roof or from the side. The vehicle may be completely de-roofed by first removing the front and rear windscreens, if present. Rescue crews are trained to avoid breaking glass, and will try to remove the windscreens fully intact if possible. The car pillars are then cut as low as possible to door level. The last pillar to be cut is usually the one next to the occupant. Once the vehicle is de-roofed, the casualty can be lifted easily, with due attention to the spine. This method is by far the safest in terms of minimising spinal movement for the casualty, but it is also the most time consuming. It is also only applicable to vehicles in which the seat can recline (either by design or by cutting) which is not the case in single-seater vehicles or some other race vehicles.

A quicker alternative to de-roofing, and one that requires fewer personnel, is called 'flapping the roof' – a similar process to opening a can of sardines whereby the front two pairs of pillars are cut and the roof is peeled back. Another strategy that is particularly useful when the racing car is on its side involves flapping the roof sideways and down. This technique is especially beneficial when the head of the casualty is lying against the pillar closest to him.

Another technique for gaining access is through the side of the racing car. Once the side door, or doors, have been opened (forcefully or otherwise) the central pillar of the car is cut close to the roof. Intersecting cuts are then made into the chassis on either side of the central pillar, and the pillar bent down to lie flat or cut out altogether.

This 'B-Post Rip' technique is the most commonly used in racing cars, since the removal of the roof is of limited help in most situations. It gives speedy access, and has the advantage that only a minimal degree of movement of the casualty is required to facilitate extrication in the hands of experienced crews.

The Medical Rescue Unit

A paramedic or qualified doctor will probably make up the Medical Rescue Unit. In the UK, the doctor will probably be dressed in red overalls, with the paramedic in green overalls. In some instances the medical staff will travel in a separate vehicle, but they may arrive with the Race Rescue Unit. The doctor will make an assessment of the casualty on arrival and deal immediately with any life-threatening conditions. Once the casualty is stabilised, an assessment will also be made of the degree of entrapment and how rapidly the doctor wishes the casualty to be extricated.

The doctor will follow the same priorities of Airway, Breathing, and Circulation described in the earlier section. Only this time, with medical aids at hand, there will be more intervention.

Assuming you are conscious and orientated, your coherent replies to the doctor's queries will indicate that at least your airway, breathing, and circulation are intact for the moment. The doctor and an assistant will attempt to take off your helmet in a controlled manner. You will be requested not to move your head while it is being supported in a neutral position by a crew member. The chin strap will be cut or undone and the helmet removed, either from the rear or front, at all times keeping the head supported. PLEASE DO NOT INTERFERE WITH THIS IMPORTANT MANOEUVRE, EVEN THOUGH YOU THINK YOUR NECK IS OK.

A stiff collar will then be applied around your neck which will restrict your neck movements. That is exactly what it is designed to do, so do not panic. Even after this is done, a crew member will continue to support your head, and it is possible that your ears may be covered by his hands as this is being done.

At this stage, if not before, an oxygen mask may be applied to your face. These masks can be claustrophobic, but forewarned is forearmed!

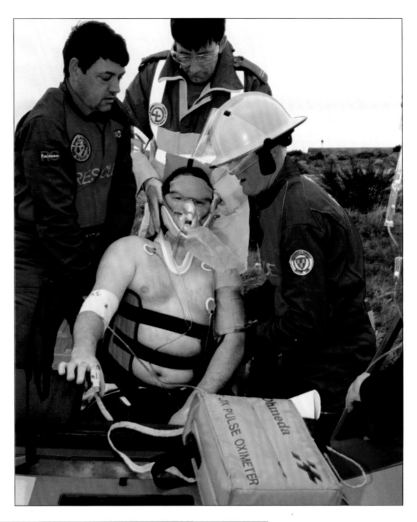

ABOVE: A de-roofed competition car with the casualty being lifted vertically using a spinal protection device. *(Roger Bell)*

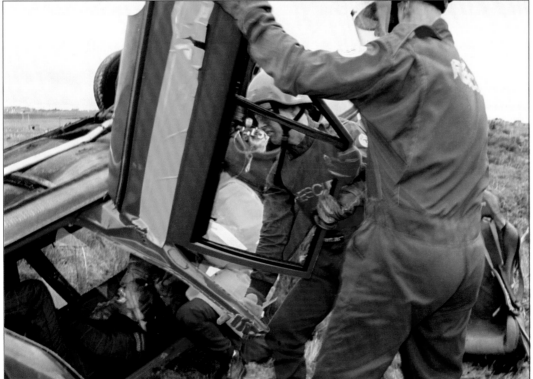

LEFT: Folding down the side of a racing car on its roof. This is a useful method of gaining access to the casualty from the side. *(Roger Bell)*

Removal of a casualty's helmet from the front while his head is being supported by a crew member. This is easier with an open-face helmet – a closed helmet may require the use of a helmet cutter, and application of a stiff collar designed to limit damage to the spinal cord if a neck fracture is present. Note that an oxygen mask has been placed on the casualty's face, and his head is still held in a neutral position. *(Roger Bell)*

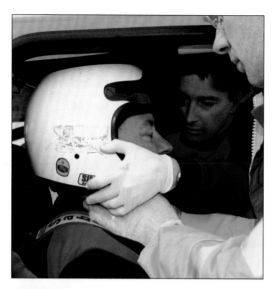
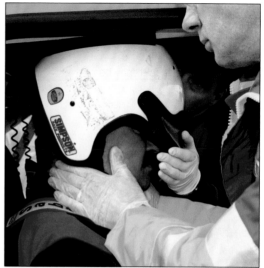
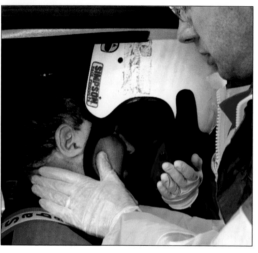
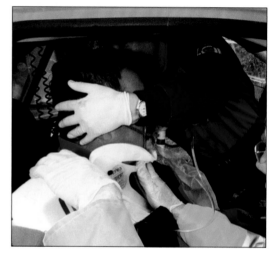
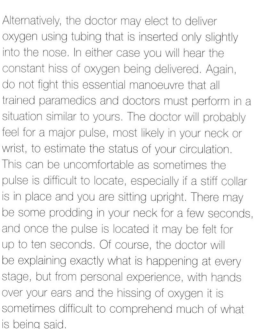

Alternatively, the doctor may elect to deliver oxygen using tubing that is inserted only slightly into the nose. In either case you will hear the constant hiss of oxygen being delivered. Again, do not fight this essential manoeuvre that all trained paramedics and doctors must perform in a situation similar to yours. The doctor will probably feel for a major pulse, most likely in your neck or wrist, to estimate the status of your circulation. This can be uncomfortable as sometimes the pulse is difficult to locate, especially if a stiff collar is in place and you are sitting upright. There may be some prodding in your neck for a few seconds, and once the pulse is located it may be felt for up to ten seconds. Of course, the doctor will be explaining exactly what is happening at every stage, but from personal experience, with hands over your ears and the hissing of oxygen it is sometimes difficult to comprehend much of what is being said.

The doctor or paramedic may try to insert an intravenous line into your arm. Again, this practice is essential, as fluids have to be provided to someone in your circumstances. The location of choice is on the inside of your elbow. Insertion may first involve cutting your race suit arm to gain access. A tourniquet will then be applied to your upper arm to 'raise a vein' and the line inserted with a sharp needle. Most people feel only a jab when the line is inserted. The line will then be taped down and a flat board strapped to your arm in some circumstances. This board prevents you from bending your elbow and kinking the line as fluids run into you.

There are possible life-threatening emergencies that trained medical staff must check for and exclude before considering you sufficiently stable for extrication. This involves examining your chest, best done by cutting off your race suit and underwear with heavy-duty scissors. The doctor may examine you using a stethoscope. While the doctor listens to your heart and lungs using a stethoscope, try not to speak to him. Instead, take in normal breaths with your mouth open. Part of the chest examination will involve carefully feeling your chest wall. Do let the doctor know what part is tender, if any, as this will help him focus on that particular area.

At some point a light may be shone into your eyes to check the size of your pupils. This gives the doctor an idea of whether any severe internal head damage is present. To make sure your spine has not been damaged, you will probably be asked if you have any weaknesses or 'pins and needles' feeling in your arms or legs. You may also be asked to move your toes or fingers to make sure the nerves are intact.

Some medical equipment may well be attached to monitor you as you are being extricated or transferred. A blood-pressure cuff to your upper arm and an oxygen saturation monitor on one of your fingers are commonly used. Also, if the doctor feels it appropriate, he may attach three heart leads to your chest wall to record your heart's electric activity. This may be necessary if you have suffered a heavy front-end impact, or complain of pain in the front of your chest wall, or if it is suspected that you have fractured your breastbone.

Pain relief

Strong painkillers, such as morphine, may also be given through the intravenous line, but only by an attending doctor or paramedic. Usually within several seconds of receiving a morphine-based drug, some people encounter a tingling sensation lasting seconds over most of their body. Some also experience nausea and vomiting. The drug itself is a potent painkiller that works within minutes if administered through an intravenous line. It may, however, make you feel drowsy.

Another relatively potent painkiller is Entonox, a 50:50 mixture of oxygen and nitrous oxide (also known as 'laughing gas'). It is delivered through a special demand valve that requires a good seal around the mouth and fairly deep breathing to open the valve. If the doctor suspects a skull fracture or a pneumothorax (air in the chest but outside the lung), then Entonox is not suitable. An advantage of Entonox is that it does not require a doctor to provide it.

Occasionally the doctor may choose to infiltrate local anaesthetic around a large nerve to numb the affected area. An example is a pain from a fractured thighbone, which can be dulled with a quick and often painless injection close to the femoral nerve in the groin. This injection is useful before putting the leg into a splint, and such a technique is commonly used by doctors covering motorcycling events, where such an injury is relatively common.

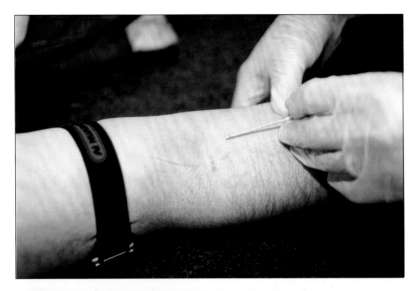

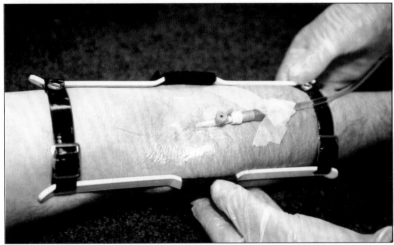

Extrication

The speed and method of removal is dictated largely by your condition and any surrounding risks. Clearly, if there is a life-threatening emergency, such as a fire, that calls for immediate removal, then you will be extricated with speed but in a controlled manner to prevent further injury. In this situation the decision to evacuate immediately is made by the doctor or paramedic who will probably support your neck and head during the extrication process. This is known as the scoop and run decision, where it is felt that, on balance, you will fare better if removed from immediate danger even though it means a risk of injury to your neck or spine.

In other situations, almost every trapped casualty will be removed with neck protection (as described earlier) and using devices designed to protect the spine. Rescue and medical teams constantly practise all forms of removal using available protection devices in various scenarios until every procedure is conducted smoothly.

ABOVE: Insertion of an intravenous line into a vein in the arm. A tourniquet, which is removed once the line is in place, can be seen on the upper arm. The second photo shows the arm being splinted and the line secured. *(Roger Bell)*

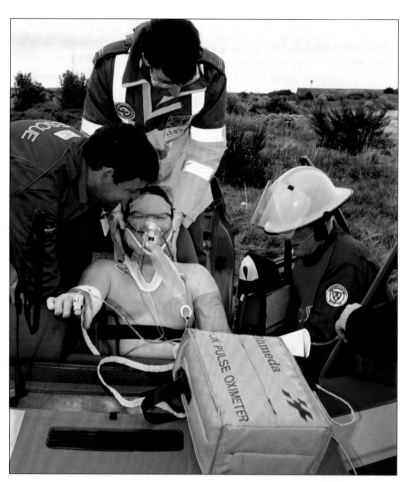

Spinal extrication devices include names such as KED, TED, and RED. They all have a similar purpose, which is to immobilise and splint your spine while moving you. The use of such devices is now mandatory for FIA events.

Applying a spinal extrication device involves teamwork and practice. Most of all, it requires cooperation from the casualty who may or may not think the procedure is necessary. As the device is being applied you will be asked to move in your seat while at all times keeping the profile of your spine unchanged. The devices also have straps that need to be fairly tight to prevent slippage when extricating. Let the teams know if the straps are too constrictive or painful as some are tightened in the crutch area.

An attempt will be made to lift you in one clean movement and without bending your back. DO NOT TRY TO HELP THE RESCUE CREW AT THIS MOMENT.

Once you have been removed from the vehicle, you will be lowered on to a long board and strapped tightly for transfer. At this point your head may be fully immobilised using head blocks and a strap across your forehead. The spinal board is exceedingly hard and uncomfortable and has been known to cause pressure sores in casualties within as little as 20 minutes.

The purpose of the long board is to facilitate

ABOVE: A casualty being stabilised while still trapped. Heart monitoring leads, an oxygen saturation probe, and a blood-pressure cuff are seen attached to the casualty, whose clothes have been cut off. It is evident that within a short time a lot of equipment, largely foreign to the casualty, will be used in a relatively confined space. *(Roger Bell)*

RIGHT: A KED, which has a supporting head cushion and straps for tightening around the chest and crutch. *(Ferno)*

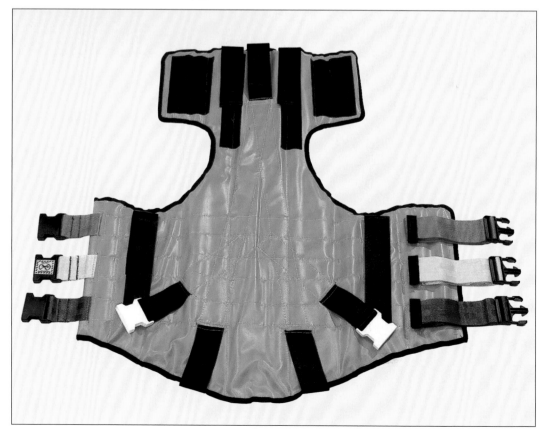

transfer on to a vacuum mattress, so you should not be on the board for more than a few minutes. Transfer on to the mattress is a single coordinated movement that assumes full cooperation from the casualty. Once placed on the vacuum mattress, air will be sucked out of the device, which then moulds itself fully around the body. The vacuum mattress is extremely effective and almost rock-hard when fully deflated. It completely immobilises you, and it can be uncomfortable on long journeys. In some cases, there may be no vacuum mattress, and transport will be on a spinal board. The spinal board may also be used from race meetings where the journey time to hospital is short, in order to facilitate rapid transfer to hospital, rather than spending time at the scene transferring the patient from one device to another. If this is the case, please do let the attending staff know if you are in pain from the area of your body in contact with the board.

In some circumstances it will be difficult to transfer a seriously injured casualty on a spinal board owing to uneven, rough ground or steep banks. Scoop stretchers allow casualty transport over such terrain but offer less protection for the spine as the weight of the casualty makes the stretcher flex. A rather painful complication of scoop stretchers is nipping of skin as the stretcher is applied or set down.

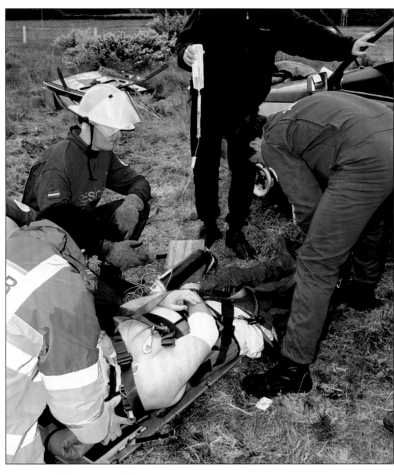

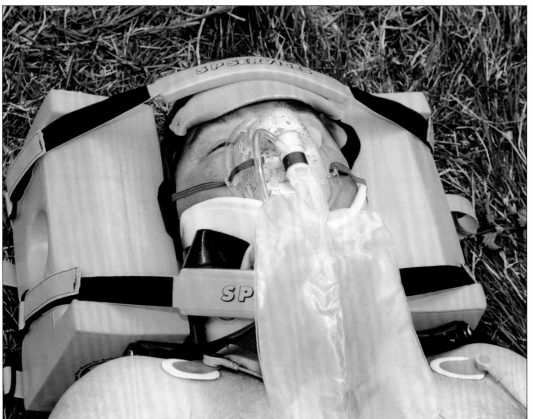

ABOVE AND LEFT: A long board with the casualty strapped tightly in ready for transfer. The head has been fully immobilised using head blocks and a Velcro-based strap across the forehead. *(Roger Bell)*

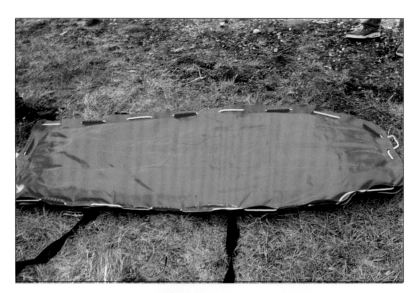

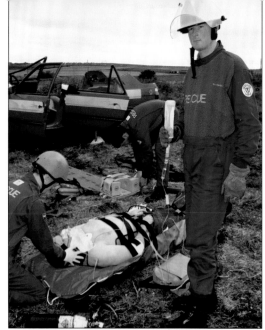

ABOVE LEFT AND RIGHT: A vacuum mattress before use, and with the casualty strapped in. *(Roger Bell)*

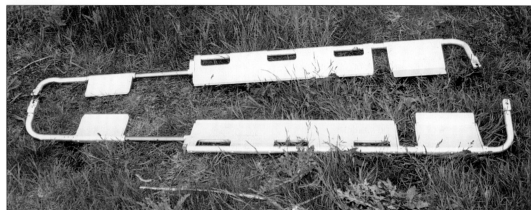

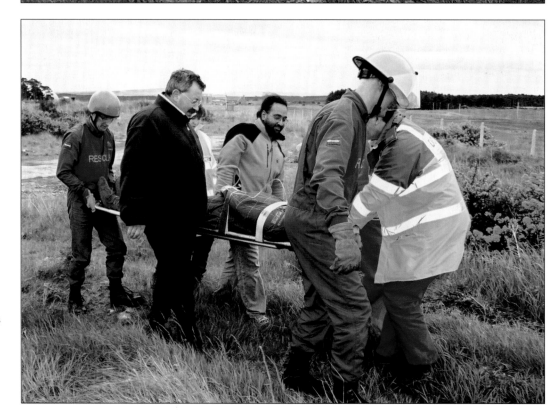

CENTRE AND RIGHT: The two halves of a scoop stretcher. This is useful for steep inclines or rough terrain, as long as the casualty is strapped on as shown in the second photo. *(Roger Bell)*

Where do you go?

In most speed and race events you will be transported to the ambulance which will then proceed to the local hospital or the circuit medical centre, depending on available resources. In some cases, such as rallies, the Rescue Unit may have to transfer you to a pre-determined rendezvous point where an ambulance may be waiting. In other cases, helicopter evacuation to hospital may be the fastest and most appropriate, especially if one is on stand-by or has been scrambled because of the nature and severity of the injuries.

Evacuation to the hospital is no fun if you are in pain, strapped tightly to a spinal board or vacuum mattress and cannot move your head even in the slightest. To make matters worse, you may have a tendency to motion sickness or are reacting to the analgesic and are feeling nauseous. Do let the staff know if you are feeling sick, as they may have to undo the head straps and support your head in readiness. They may also be able to give you some medication through a drip to reduce the sensation. Being sick while lying immobilised face up is not the greatest feeling!

Helicopter evacuation poses its own problems, and a high degree of safety precaution is essential. When Didier Pironi, the Formula 1 Ferrari driver, was being transferred to the race helicopter following his massive crash in Hockenheim in 1982 that ended his racing career, an umbrella was being used to protect his body from heavy

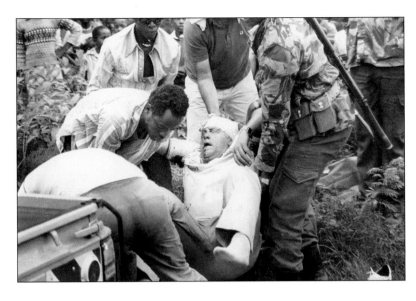

rain. As the stretcher party approached the helicopter the top of the umbrella caught the main rotor blades damaging them. The bearer was considered lucky not to have been decapitated!

During helicopter transfer, noise levels and vibration are usually very high and occasionally uncomfortable. If not already applied, ask for ear defenders. It may be useful to have predetermined signals ready for use in case you experience increasing pain and discomfort. Another potential problem is to do with flicker from the rotors. While it can very rarely lead to fits, it may more commonly cause vertigo.

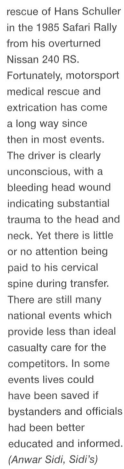

ABOVE AND LEFT: The rescue of Hans Schuller in the 1985 Safari Rally from his overturned Nissan 240 RS. Fortunately, motorsport medical rescue and extrication has come a long way since then in most events. The driver is clearly unconscious, with a bleeding head wound indicating substantial trauma to the head and neck. Yet there is little or no attention being paid to his cervical spine during transfer. There are still many national events which provide less than ideal casualty care for the competitors. In some events lives could have been saved if bystanders and officials had been better educated and informed. (Anwar Sidi, Sidi's)

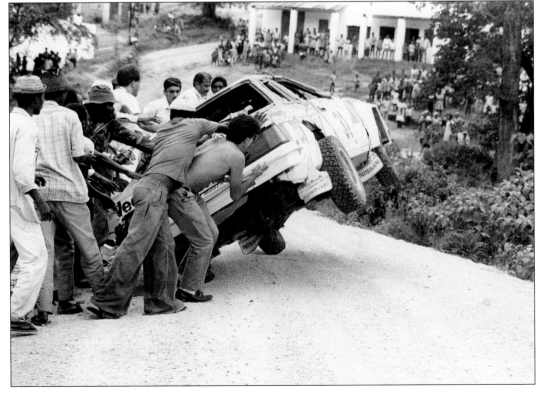

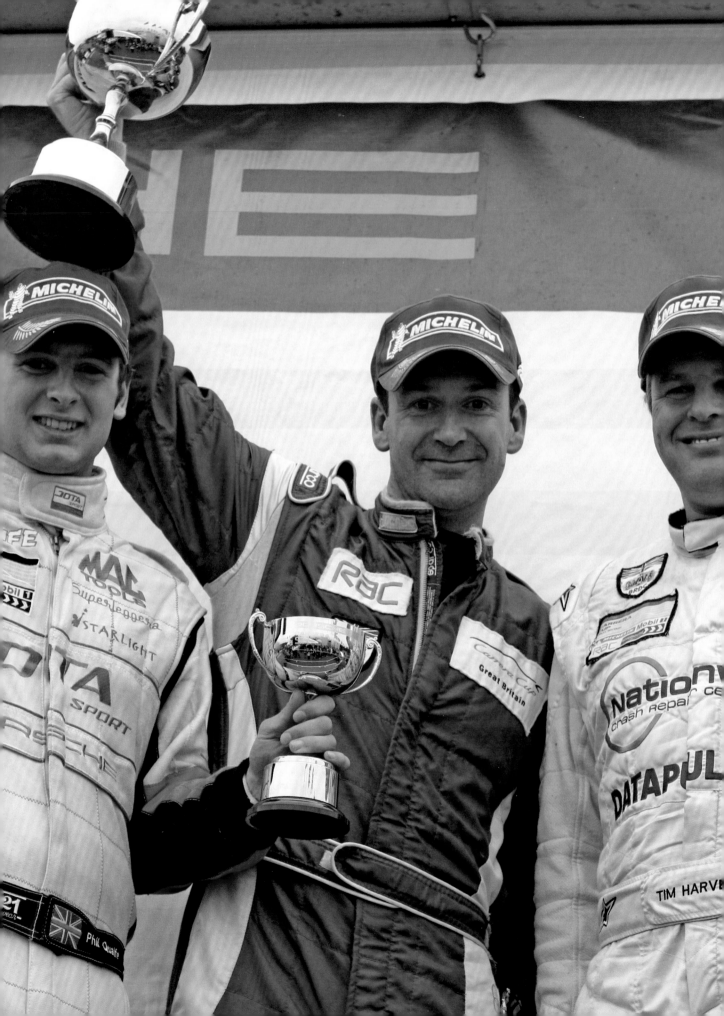

13

Getting a licence to race

The FIA (Fédération Internationale de l'Automobile) based in Geneva, Switzerland, is the leading international body that makes and enforces rules relating to automobile competitions. The rules are drawn up in a document called the International Sporting Code which, along with its appendices, can be viewed on the FIA's website (www.fia.com) or in the *FIA Yearbook*. Each country taking part in motorsport has a club or federation known as an ASN (National Automobile Club) that can affiliate itself to the FIA. The ASN is then bound by the rules of the Code and enforces them at national level. In the British Isles (excluding the Republic of Ireland) the ASN is the MSA (Motor Sports Association) based at Colnbrook, England. Its website is www.msauk.org.

Each ASN may draw up its own regulations. The MSA's regulations can be found in the *MSA Competitors' Yearbook* (known as 'The Blue Book'). Although they may be worded differently they all comply more or less with the Code issued by the FIA. In the UK the regulations are also reviewed by the British government's Office of Fair Trading to make sure the practices are satisfactory.

Who can and cannot race?

First, check with your ASN about age eligibility, as there are certain minimum age limits that apply depending upon the type of event entered.

Also, competing in motorsport events can be precluded by some medical conditions. For FIA international status events these include instances where limb movement is restricted by more than 50%; where there have been amputations (except where fingers are lost but grip function in both

hands is retained); where orthopaedic prostheses are used (the resulting function being not normal or near normal); and where epilepsy exists and is still under treatment, or where there is an associated behavioural affect. Many ASNs, including the MSA, may take a more lenient approach, so it is worth checking with your local ASN if you are not sure.

Other conditions may require a medical assessment by someone approved by the ASN before a licence can be issued. These include insulin-dependent diabetes, heart valve problems, and angina. Those who have had a heart attack or have suffered from other heart conditions, have orthopaedic prostheses, have limited hand movement or have existing psychiatric conditions are also assessed individually.

If you are in doubt about an existing medical condition, contact your ASN which may have a specialist advisory panel to help. Remember, ASNs do not set out to fail everyone who applies, and they will work with you to reach, it is hoped, a favourable decision.

The medical examination

It goes without saying that motorsport can be dangerous, and racing places a great strain on the system. High body-temperature, vehicle vibration, muscular and emotional stress all have to be contended with. Heart rates close to 200 beats per minute have been recorded even in professional drivers, and they are far fitter than amateur competitors. These stresses are tolerated better if you are mentally relaxed, well hydrated, and physically fit. But, for example, anyone with a hidden heart complaint

OPPOSITE: Carrera Cup drivers celebrating on the podium. Every driver no matter how prominent started their career at club level. *(Mike Gibbon, MVG Photographic)*

would be unlikely to withstand them and might suffer irreversible damage, or even death, while competing. The medical examination is designed to detect such weaknesses so that they can be given early treatment and, it is hoped, thereby restoring the chance to race. I say this as a doctor performing routine driver medicals, and as a driver who receives medical examinations. In my experience there is little that will fail someone outright that he or she does not already know about. Dr R. S. Jutley

Appendix L of the International Sporting Code clearly states the need for a medical examination to obtain an international licence from the ASN, and an annual one thereafter. It is no concern of

the FIA how or to whom an ASN issues licences for events at national level, as these events do not fall within FIA jurisdiction. Each ASN is entitled to apply its own rules and some are stricter than others. In Britain this regulation is met by requesting all applicants to complete an annual self-declaration of medical fitness. A medical examination and eye test is recommended if the applicant has not had either of these recently. Certain applicants, such as those applying for a Car, Truck or Kart licence, over the age of 18, must have a medical examination. This may be followed by an annual self-declaration until age 45, after which competitors must pass a medical examination each year.

Although the format of the medical examination

Section 3 – Your doctor's medical report on you

To your doctor
Please read the enclosed Competition Licence Notes before filling in this section for your patient whose name is on the front of this form.

1. Your practice stamp (together with your name and qualifications):

2. Are you the applicant's usual doctor?   Yes ☐   No ☐

3. Is there any evidence of abnormality of the heart or cardiovascular system?   Yes ☐ No ☐
If 'Yes', give details below.

If the applicant is 45 or over and applying for an international licence, we need a written report on a stress-related ECG (see note R7).

4. Is there any evidence of a physical or mental condition (past or present) which could, in your opinion, prevent the applicant from holding a competition licence for motor sport?   Yes ☐ No ☐
If 'Yes', give details below.

5. Does the applicant have any physical abnormality or restriction of movement in the arms or legs?   Yes ☐ No ☐
If 'Yes', give details below.

6. Vision – Uncorrected   R eye [/]   L eye [/]
   Corrected   R eye [/]   L eye [/]

   Vision with both eyes open (wearing corrective lenses if necessary) (see note CA26):   [/]
   Field of vision: [ ]

   Is the applicant's colour vision normal?   Yes ☐ No ☐
   If 'No', please give details below.

7. Blood pressure: [/]

8. Is the urine analysis normal?   Yes ☐ No ☐
If 'No', please give details below.

This is to certify that I have examined the applicant in line with this form and the enclosed notes.

Your doctor's signature: **Date of examination:**

RIGHT: The MSA Annual Medical Form that covers the medical examination regulations laid down by the FIA.

may vary from country to country, for international licences the FIA has stipulated the minimum requirements for each examination. Each applicant must have an eyesight test and orthopaedic examination (essentially looking at their limbs and spine functions). Also, those aged 45 and over must have a stress ECG performed to ensure there are no heart problems. This test involves the use of a treadmill in accordance with a set protocol over a specified time. The results of a stress ECG are valid for two years. Some national authorities may also insist on details of blood groups for each applicant, along with urine tests.

Medical regulations change all the time to allow for individual cases. It will be worth asking your local ASN about any new rules that may affect you. For example, the MSA has amended its regulations regarding eyesight standards after consulting with specialists to allow many competitors with monocular vision to compete.

Disabled drivers

Disabled drivers in motor sport, although uncommon, are not entirely unheard of. The Australian Mark Pope who, sadly, was rendered paraplegic by a motocross accident when he was 16, has not only competed in the Paralympics but has driven in rallies, sometimes finishing as high as second position in his class. Another example is Britain's David Butler, a triple amputee, who has qualified for full Race and Rally licences. The FIA does issue special licences for drivers who have a congenital or acquired handicap as long as certain criteria are met. For example, applicants must have a full medical evaluation of their disabilities, and they must modify their vehicles as indicated by the ASN. An evaluation must also be made of their ability to extract themselves from an automobile in an emergency situation. The rules set out by the FIA state: '... he must move from a sitting to a standing position, turn easily over both ways; must be able to extricate himself vertically using an arm, and in the same way be able to exit laterally.'

There are special competition rules for handicapped drivers and these depend largely on a competitor's former and current driving skills. It is best to check with the ASN whether any events are running for handicapped drivers or whether you qualify to compete alongside non-handicapped drivers. The latter will depend upon your skills, and requires assessment by the FIA Medical Commission and Circuits and Safety Commission.

Special organisations have been established to represent disabled drivers wishing to compete in motorsport. One of these is the British Motorsport Association for the Disabled (BMSAD). Set up in 1987, it has helped over 100 competitors gain the right to compete in various motorsport events.

Doping

The FIA and all affiliated organisations are clear on their policy with regard to doping. International competitors found to test positive in FIA-sanctioned events are reported either directly or indirectly to the President of the FIA. Offences that are serious can be judged directly by the FIA without involvement of the local ASN. In national events, however, the ASN may deal with the matter entirely.

The MSA randomly tests for drugs and alcohol, and any competitor testing positive is reported to the MSA. If the test results are upheld they will be asked to appear before an MSA tribunal and they will be reported to the Sports Council.

The International Olympic Committee (IOC) regularly reviews the list of substances and methods open to abuse. The updates may be viewed on the FIA website. Motorsport bodies generally use the IOC list of banned substances, with the important addition of alcohol. It is worth paying the site a visit to find out what may happen if you are requested to provide a sample for analysis. Your ASN or the FIA may request samples. The President of the FIA also has the authority to request spot checks not only during competitions but also at any time. Any competitor failing to comply will be subject to sanctions.

Some general advice

Along with what the FIA states in its regulations, the following general advice is also useful.

You should know your blood group and tetanus status. If you have not been immunised against tetanus you are strongly advised to have this done. Competitors with life-threatening allergies, especially to antibiotics, should wear identity tags detailing the allergy, and it is recommended that you tell the event medical officer of your condition before competing. The same advice applies to asthmatics and those who require special medical treatment. If you are in any doubt about your pre-existing condition, then early liaison with the event doctor will guard against any problems should an emergency arise.

All motorsport bodies advise against chewing gum while racing as this could become caught in the throat and cause an airway blockage. For the same reason false dentures should be removed.

Appendices

References

Alford, C. et al 'The Effects of Red Bull Energy Drink on Human Performance and Mood', *Amino Acids* 2001; 21:139-150.

Almond, L. & Newberry, I. 'The importance of physical activity in weight management', *Obesity in Practice*, 2:10-12; 2000.

Allied Dunbar National Fitness Survey – Main Findings, London: Sports Council and Health Education Authority, 1992.

Armstrong et al 'Urinary Indices of Hydration Status', *International Journal of Sports Nutrition* 1994; 4:265-79.

Bean, Anita *The Complete Guide to Sports Nutrition* (3rd edition), A. & C. Black, London, 2000.

Bertrand, C., Keromes, A., Lemeunier, B. F., Meistelmann, C., Prieur, C. & Richalet, J. P. 'Physiologie des Sports Mécanques', 1st International Congress of Sport Automobile, Marseilles, 1983 in *Life at the Limit*, Sid Watkins, Macmillan Publishers, London, 1996.

Brukner, P. & Khan, K. *Clinical Sports Medicine*, McGraw-Hill Company, Australia, 2000.

Cooper, K. H. 'A means of assessing maximum oxygen uptake', *Journal of the American Medical Association*, 1968; 203:201-204.

Kay, D., Taaffe, D. R. & Marino, F. E. 'Whole-body pre-cooling and heat storage during self-paced cycling performance in warm humid conditions', *Journal of Sports Sciences*, 17: 937-944.

Kline, G., Pocari, J., Hintermeister, R., Freedson, P., Ward, A., McCarron, R., Ross, J. & Rippe, J. 'Estimation of VO$_2$max from a one-mile track walk, gender, age, and body weight'. *Medicine and Science in Sports and Exercise*, 1987; 19:253-259.

Lakka, T., Venalainen, J., Rauramaa, R., Salonen, R., Tuomilehto, J. & Salonen, J. 'Relation of leisure-time physical activity and cardiorespiratory fitness to the risk of acute myocardial infarction in men', *New England Journal of Medicine*, 1994; 330:1549-1554.

Mahieu, N., et al 'Effect of Static and Ballistic Stretching on the Muscle-Tendon Tissue Properties', *Medicine and Science in Sports and Exercise*, 2007; 39(3): 494-501.

Managing Weight, A workbook for health and other professionals, Health Education Authority, London, 1998.

McLatchie, G. *ABC of Sports Medicine*, BMJ Publishing, London, 2000.

McMillian, D., et al 'Dynamic Versus Static-Stretching Warm Up: The Effect on Power and Agility Performance', *Journal of Strength and Conditioning Research*, 2006; 20(3): 492-499.

McMorris, T., Swain, J., Lauder, M., Smith, N. & Kelly, J. 'Warm-up prior to undertaking a dynamic psychomotor task: does it aid performance?', *J. Sports Med. Phys. Fitness*, 2006; 46(2):328-34.

Orlick, T. *In Pursuit of Excellence: How to win in sport and life through mental training*, Human Kinetics, Champaign, 2000.

Rasch, W. & Cabanac, M. 'Selective brain cooling is affected by wearing headgear during exercise', *Journal of Applied Physiology* 1993; 74:1229.

Rolls, B. T., et al 'Thirst following water deprivation in humans', *American Journal of Physiology* 1980; 239:476.

Sharkey, B. J. *Fitness and Health* (4th edition), Human Kinetics, Champaign, 1997.

Smith, J. F., Bishop, P. A., Ellis, L., Conerly, M. D. & Mansfield, E. R. 'Exercise intensity increased by addition of handheld weights to rebounding exercise', *J. Cardiopulm. Rehabil.*; 15:34-8.

Stephens, J., et al 'Lengthening the Hamstring Muscles Without Stretching Using "Awareness Through Movement"', *Physical Therapy* 2006; 86:1641-1650.

Watkins, Sid, *Life at the Limit*, Macmillan Publishers, London, 1996.

Willardson, J. M. 'Core stability training: applications to sports conditioning programs', *J. Strength Cond. Res.* 2007; 21(3):979-85.

Woods, K., Bishop, P. & Jones, E. 'Warm-up and stretching in the prevention of muscular injury', *Sports Med.* 2007; 37(12):1089-99.

World Health Organisation 'Obesity – promoting and managing the global epidemic', Report of a WHO consultation on obesity, Geneva, 1998.

The contributors

Chris Blythin MSCP, BSc (Hons)

Chris graduated as a physiotherapist from the University of Southampton in 2002. Since then he has worked in a variety of settings, including sports injury clinics, the sports field, the NHS, and the fitness testing lab. He went on to train in Kinetic Control, soft tissue release, manipulation, muscle energy techniques, and in 2006 passed the Society of Orthopaedic Medicine exam. A keen endurance athlete himself, Chris has always focused on the importance of prevention in preference to cure. Working with votwo, Chris has used his deep understanding of ergonomics and injury management to help racing drivers and endurance athletes rehabilitate back to full fitness. Chris has often been concerned at the tendency for some racing drivers to neglect flexibility work. The effects of this have seemed to be all too apparent, and so he has targeted the flexibility chapter at specifically improving flexibility in the driving position.

Barbara Cox

Barbara Cox is a highly regarded nutritionist and CEO of Nutrichef Ltd, a healthy meal delivery company. She became passionate about the importance of eating healthily during an eight-year stay in Japan, a country renowned for its low levels of obesity, cancer, and heart disease. Through her consultations with Nutrichef customers across the UK, Barbara advises people with a range of concerns, including people wishing to lose weight, athletes training for sports events or people who simply want to find out what it means to eat healthily. Barbara writes articles on nutrition for a variety of publications and is a regional winner of Entrepreneur of the Year.

Dr Jonathan Whelan BM, BSc (Hons), FRCA, DIPIMC, RCS(Ed)

Dr Whelan is an MSA-registered anaesthetist who undertakes medical cover for the British Automobile Racing Club (BARC) and other racing clubs across the UK. He is also the Chief Medical Officer at Thruxton Circuit in Hampshire. He provides medical cover for large events such as World Superbikes and British Touring Cars.

Mike Garth

Mike Garth helps karters, racing drivers, and motorcycle racers perform better by maximising their mental approach. An ex-circuit racer, Mike was Head of R&D at Reynard Motorsport, helping the company win seven straight Champ Car Drivers' and Constructors' World Series Championships, before moving on to the Race and Test engineering teams at Toyota F1. The realisation that racing performance was mostly a human issue rather than a technical one lead Mike to further training. Now a fully accredited sport psychologist with the British Association of Sport and Exercise Sciences, Mike owns the Sun1400 performance coaching consultancy, with clients in F1, F Renault, F BMW, and all levels of British and European karting.

Bernie Shrosbree

Bernie Shrosbree is one of the most renowned fitness trainers in world motorsport. Having worked with many household names in Rallying, Formula 1, and even Olympic rowing, his level of experience in the field is second to none. With a unique background as an elite endurance athlete and Royal Marine, Bernie has a wealth of extreme experiences to draw upon that provide the foundation to his coaching style. Still an active athlete himself, Bernie can often be found kayaking, cross-country skiing, cycling or climbing with his training clients or simply for his own pleasure.

Eliot Challifour

Having graduated from the University of Bath in 2005, Eliot established the sports coaching company votwo alongside author Andy Blow. He presently works with a number of votwo's top motorsport clients, overseeing their training programmes. Additionally he has coached two age-group triathlon World Champions, and athletes who have qualified for the Hawaii Ironman. As an active athlete himself, Eliot has competed at international level in triathlon, and takes part in extreme endurance events on a regular basis.

Contributors from Fit for Motorsport, 2003

Aman Agarwal of Harvey's, Edinburgh (Turner's Construction); Bernie Shrosbree, ex-Human Performance Manager, Renault F1; Colin Wilson of the MSA, Crowood Press; Dr David Cranston; Dr John Harrington, Chief Medical Officer, Speyside Rally, Snowman Rally, and Colin McRae Forest Stages; Dr Matt Smith; Dr Rob Johnston; Fiona Walsh; Flora Myer; Granite City Rescue crew (Dave 'Sid' Simpson, Crew Chief, Graham Bruce, Stu Castleton, Steve Wright, Anne-Marie Cassidy, Cpl Roger 'Dinger' Bell); Human Kinetics; Iain McPherson; Jan Gibbon; Jim Moodie; John Hardaker; Ken Walker, ex-Chairman of the MSA medical advisory committee; Louise Aitken-Walker MBE; Lynne Howe-Green; Martin Holmes Rallying (Maurice Selden and Martin Holmes); McKlein (Colin McMaster); McRaes (Jim McRae and Colin McRae MBE – *R.I.P.*); MVG Photographic (Mike Gibbon); Naveed Iqbal of www.worldrallying.com; Next Generation Clubs and Life Fitness (David Lloyd, Patrick Coote, Malcolm McPhail); Hayleigh Maxfield; Paul Lewis in Aberdeen for legal advice; Prof Sid Watkins; Quotronics Systems (Dr David Nelson); Renault Formula 1 (Sarah Blackham and the PR staff); Robbie Head of Channel 4 WRC; Roy Smith and Jamie Smith for loan of their rally car; Sarah Christofi and Barbara Serhant of Red Bull; Sarah Hughes for IT skills; Servier Laboratories Limited; Shire Rescue Crew (Brian Hatton and Steve); Sidi's Photography, Kenya (Anwar Sidi); Tina Biddlecombe; Victor Morgan of VM Sports Agencies.

Finally, I am grateful to my wife, Anita Kaur Jutley, for her tireless support in all aspects, and I apologise to all those who I may have forgotten to thank.

Dr R. S. Jutley

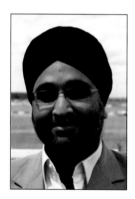

Dr R. S. Jutley

Andy Blow

Author's notes ...

It is almost seven years since *Fit for Motorsport*, the precursor of this book, was launched with Professor Sid Watkins at the world's largest motorsport gathering, the *Autosport* Show at the National Exhibition Centre in Birmingham. It was received enthusiastically, with reviews in respected publications, such as the *Independent on Sunday*. Pleasingly, all printed copies were sold out within a few years. In fact, much to my amusement, I ran out of personal copies when the time came to give reference copies to invited co-authors for the reworking of the second edition. The ones available were selling in the USA at several times the original price. This edition promises even more. There are more quotes from leading drivers, chapters rewritten by experts, and the exercise routines and advice have been brought up to date. The most important change has been the invitation of a co-author, Andy Blow – a well-known personality in motorsport human performance.

Andy started his career as a sports scientist at the Benetton, later Renault F1, Human Performance Centre under the guidance of top motorsport fitness trainer Bernie Shrosbree – who contributed substantially to *Fit For Motorsport*. Andy worked with world-class drivers such as Giancarlo Fisichella, Mark Webber, Alex Wurz, Fernando Alonso, and Jenson Button, amongst others. He closely observed the way that these professionals prepared for their high-pressure, high-profile job driving some of the fastest race cars available, thus gaining invaluable insight into the incredible physical and mental demands that motorsport places on drivers. Andy's contributions are invaluable and I am delighted to have him, and his team of professionals at votwo, on board.

Dr R. S. Jutley BMedSci (Hon), MB, ChB, DM, FRCSGlas (C-Th)

The technology on today's amateur race cars is often filtered down from the higher echelons of the sport, such as the WRC or F1 arenas. I firmly believe that the exact training techniques and methods that put drivers of these top machines at the pinnacle of motorsport can also be filtered down to competitors at any level. My own background, competing in triathlon and other endurance competitions, has also broadened my understanding of training, nutrition, and preparation for competition in extreme environments – some as extreme as the Ironman events. Aspects of this book, therefore, aim to consolidate my professional and practical sporting experiences into accessible advice for those wishing to improve their own physical and mental performance in motorsport. Working with Dr Jutley on the project has been hugely rewarding, as his vast medical knowledge and real-life experiences in the rallying world have allowed us to share ideas and produce something that is, we hope, greater than the sum of its parts.

Andy Blow BSc (Hon)

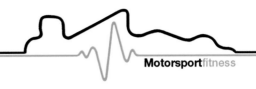

Index